Introductory Guide to Cardiac Catheterization

Second Edition

Arman T. Askari, MD, FACC
Clinical Associate Professor of Medicine
Case Western Reserve University, Attending Cardiologist
Harrington–McLaughlin Heart & Vascular Institute
University Hospitals Case Medical Center
Cleveland, Ohio

Mehdi H. Shishehbor, DO, MPH
Staff, Vascular Medicine & Interventional Cardiology
Heart & Vascular Institute Cleveland Clinic
Cleveland, Ohio

Adrian W. Messerli, MD, FACC, FSCAI
Co-Director, Cardiac Catheterization Laboratory
St. Joseph Hospital
Lexington, Kentucky

Ronnier J. Aviles, MD, FACC
Staff Interventional Cardiologist
Overlake Hospital Medical Center
Investigator, Hope Heart Institute
Bellevue, Washington

Wolters Kluwer | Lippincott Williams & Wilkins
Health
Philadelphia • Baltimore • New York • London
Buenos Aires • Hong Kong • Sydney • Tokyo

Acquisitions Editor: Frances R. DeStefano
Product Manager: Leanne McMillan
Production Manager: Bridgett Dougherty
Senior Manufacturing Manager: Benjamin Rivera
Marketing Manager: Kimberly Schonberger
Design Coordinator: Teresa Mallon
Production Service: MPS Limited, A Macmillan Company

© 2011 by LIPPINCOTT WILLIAMS & WILKINS, a WOLTERS KLUWER business
Two Commerce Square
2001 Market Street
Philadelphia, PA 19103, USA
LWW.com

Printed in China

Library of Congress Cataloging-in-Publication Data

Introductory guide to cardiac catheterization/[edited by] Arman T. Askari ... [et al.].—2nd ed.
    p. ; cm.
    Includes bibliographical references and index.
    Summary: "The staff in every catheterization laboratory in the world participates in some form of hazing. Although largely benign and expected, this ritual can place even more stress on an already unsettled and insecure newcomer. The first edition of this manual was spearheaded by cardiology fellows who remembered well what it was like to enter the cath lab for the first time. Now, several years later, these 'hazees' have in many cases become the 'hazers' but the additional experience and responsibility has allowed for a more comprehensive and updated manual.Our goal is to produce a thoroughly practical and easily accessible manual for physicians, physicians-in-training, nurses, cath lab x-ray techs, mid-level providers and students. Since we have been subjected to years of questions, first from our mentors and now from our students, we are acutely familiar with the most pertinent and necessary data for any student no matter the level of training. The manual remains specifically designed with an easy-to-read format that includes highlighted 'pearls,' updated American College of Cardiology/American Heart Association (ACC/AHA) guidelines, numerous visuals including carefully delineated schematics of standard coronary projections, and special 'troubleshooting' notes that provide potential solutions for frequently encountered problems"—Provided by publisher.
    ISBN-13: 978-1-60547-885-2 (alk. paper)
    ISBN-10: 1-60547-885-7 (alk. paper)
    1. Cardiac catheterization—Handbooks, manuals, etc. I. Askari, Arman T.
    [DNLM: 1. Heart Catheterization—methods. 2. Coronary Angiography—methods. WG 141.5.C2 I615 2011]
    RC683.5.C25I588 2011
    616.1'20754—dc22

                                                                                           2010021076

To purchase additional copies of this book, call our customer service department at (800) 638-3030 or fax orders to (301) 223-2320. International customers should call (301) 223-2300.

Visit Lippincott Williams & Wilkins on the Internet at LWW.com. Lippincott Williams & Wilkins customer service representatives are available from 8:30 am to 6 pm, EST.

CCS0810

*To our families for their continuous and faithful support . . .
Jamie, Alexa, Amanda, Jacob, Ali, Houri, Andrea, Zakarias, Emily, Mia, Katie, Marco, Jennifer, and Joshua.*

CONTENTS

FOREWORD TO THE FIRST EDITION

Consider you are a novice to the catheterization laboratory. Apparently, you got hold of *Introductory Guide to Cardiac Catheterization*. Now, all you have to do is retire for an afternoon and study it. You will still be a novice, but you will be an enlightened and knowledgeable novice.

The authors, primarily cardiology fellows instrumental for the content and format of the manual, look at the challenging, sometimes frustrating, but mostly gratifying work in the cardiac catheterization laboratory from the front end. I look at it from the back end, with the perspective of a lifelong career, and I see things exactly as they do. This comes as close as anything to guaranteeing that the content of this book is intelligible, valuable, and lasting.

In a succinct style and a condensed format, the authors report from the scene. It is apparent that they have been in the midst of the action for a while; that they have been wide awake while being there; and that they have been blessed with the particular talent to grasp things, weigh them, and convey them. Of course, the sedimented experiences of the senior authors transpire here and there, particularly when pearls are pointed out that give away the old crack. For instance, the importance of the conus branch of the right coronary artery is highlighted. The conus branch is often missed when it takes off separately from the right coronary artery, and it may be the only contributor to an occluded left anterior descending coronary artery. Or it is recommended to keep attempts to pass a stenosed aortic valve in time with systole. In diastole, it is indeed impossible to pass the valve as it is closed; trivial, but blatantly ignored by most of us.

The manual is made for readers or browsers. The readers will prevail, as this is one of those books that are hard to put down. Hence, most will start reading nonchalantly about how to prepare themselves and the patients for what has to be done in the catheterization laboratory. Then they will casually settle down more comfortably to learn all they need to learn, but not a thing more, about radiation protection and the basic material, just before diving into some tricks of the trade explained in plain words and with high-quality photographs and illustrations wherever pertinent. By now, they will be practically oblivious to what is going on around them. Only the lazy ones will skip the somewhat more demanding chapter on hemodynamics, muttering excuses such as "in my place, the computer does this." This chapter has been the kernel of the thick-belly books on cardiac catheterization of yesteryear. It still needs to be there, but it needs to be there in a lean and stripped-down version such as what is found in Chapter 6. One certainly should resist the temptation to skip the final short chapter about the aftercare, because this usually is more important for the patient than the brief intermezzo in the catheterization laboratory, most of which he or she missed anyhow.

I also recommend this compendium for cardiologists in the phase of only toying with the idea of commencing a career in the catheterization laboratory. They will be reminded that the video game–like thrill in finding the artery and being able to engage the coronary ostium in a reasonable time is but the tip of the iceberg. What lies beneath is tough, partly repetitious, and at times boring routine work with more immediate responsibility than many of us might care to bear. When pioneers like Cournand, Sones, and Judkins introduced diagnostic cardiac catheterization and Rubio-Alvarez, Rashkind, King, and Gruentzig added a therapeutic scent to it, they created a field of action for a new breed of doctor: a mixture between the internist with a big brain and the hands in the pockets and the gung-ho surgeon with big guts and the hands in everything but the pockets. *Introductory Guide to Cardiac Catheterization* will help you to find out whether you are one of that league or whether it is worth (and safe) for you to try to become one. Enjoy it!

Bernhard Meier, MD
Professor and Head of Cardiology
Swiss Cardiovascular Center Bern
University Hospital
Bern, Switzerland

FOREWORD TO THE SECOND EDITION

The trainee beginning in the cardiac catheterization laboratory (physician, nurse, tech, or PA) is faced with the daunting task of quickly assimilating a number of foreign concepts, including a new vocabulary, manual skills requiring considerable dexterity, the need to quickly translate two-dimensional images into three-dimensional anatomy and to relate these findings to the clinical condition of the person before them, all in the context of a potentially ill and vulnerable patient. For decades this has been largely practiced as an apprenticeship. Historically, however, most apprenticeships didn't have an immediate risk as harmful to the consumer (or patient) as this.

There is, therefore, a pressing need to accelerate the learning curve of the apprentice. The second edition of *Introductory Guide to Catheterization* helps achieve this goal. It succinctly presents the basic concepts and skills in a very readable fashion, from the perspective of an experienced veteran of the cardiac catheterization laboratory. Vascular access (femoral, radial, or brachial), closure, the avoidance of errors of omission (failure to find the errant high anterior right coronary artery ostium) and commission (too superior an access to the femoral artery resulting in increased risk of retroperitoneal bleed), and key hemodynamic interpretations (tips to distinguish constructive vs. restrictive pathophysiology) are all reviewed. The many illustrations and labeled angiograms are a particular strength. It can be read in reasonably short order as a prelude to stepping into the catheterization laboratory, or as a reference when one has come across or approaches an unfamiliar clinical situation.

All chapters have been meaningfully updated and new chapters on peripheral angiography and key study questions have been added.

I wish that I had access to such a text when I began my career in the cardiac catheterization laboratory nearly 30 years ago. I too readily recall not knowing what was expected of me next, not understanding why the same sequence of events wasn't pursued in every patient, and in particular why my mentor kept trying to pull the diagnostic catheterization out of the patient's groin when I was laboring to torque it into the right coronary artery (these were the days just before the routine use of vascular sheaths, and he wanted to make certain that I wouldn't inadvertently let the catheter come out of the femoral artery!). Many things have changed since then, but the basics remain.

Stephen G. Ellis, MD
Section Head of Invasive/Interventional Cardiology
Robert and Suzanne Tomsich Department of Cardiovascular Medicine
Sydell and Arnold Miller Family Heart & Vascular Institute
Cleveland Clinic
Cleveland, Ohio

PREFACE

The staff in every catheterization laboratory in the world participate in some form of hazing. Although largely benign and expected, this ritual can place even more stress on an already unsettled and insecure newcomer. The first edition of this manual was spearheaded by cardiology fellows who remembered well what it was like to enter the cath lab for the first time. Now, several years later, these "hazees" have in many cases become the "hazers," but the additional experience and responsibility have allowed for a more comprehensive and updated manual.

Our goal is to produce a thoroughly practical and easily accessible manual for physicians, physicians-in-training, nurses, cath lab x-ray techs, mid-level providers, and students. Since we have been subjected to years of questions, first from our mentors and now from our students, we are acutely familiar with the most pertinent and necessary data for any student no matter the level of training. The manual remains specifically designed with an easy-to-read format that includes highlighted "pearls," updated American College of Cardiology/American Heart Association (ACC/AHA) guidelines, numerous visuals including carefully delineated schematics of standard coronary projections, and special "troubleshooting" notes that provide potential solutions for frequently encountered problems. Also included are new chapters on peripheral angiography and study questions. The manual is intended to fit conveniently within a lab coat pocket, so that it may readily serve as a reference should a bout of hazing demand quick study!

We wish to acknowledge and thank Dr. Stephen Ellis, who spent not only hundreds of hours teaching each of the editors, but also wrote a beautiful foreword to our second edition. We remain grateful to Marion Tomasko, Suzanne Turner, Charlene Surace, and Mary Ann Citraro who worked tirelessly on the original graphics within this manual. Also, we thank once again Dr. Bernhard Meier who provided us with a wondrously supportive foreword to our first edition (enclosed). Finally, a particularly fond nod of thanks is due each of the cardiology fellows who has contributed to either edition of this manual.

We are grateful for the insightful criticisms we received from readers on our first edition, and have incorporated many suggestions into this effort. Hopefully the education provided herein is more comprehensive as a result! We value further feedback and suggestions. Please email any comments or thoughts you might have to cathmanual@gmail.com.

Adrian W. Messerli, MD

CONTRIBUTING AUTHORS

Mateen Akhtar, MD
Cardiologist
Wake Heart & Vascular Associates
Smithfield, North Carolina

Kellan E. Ashley, MD
Interventional Cardiology Fellow
Department of Cardiovascular
*   Medicine*
Cleveland Clinic
Cleveland, Ohio

Bethany A. Austin, MD
Fellow in Cardiovascular Disease
Department of Cardiovascular
*   Medicine*
Cleveland Clinic
Cleveland, Ohio

Sorin J. Brener, MD
Professor of Medicine
Department of Medicine
Ohio State University
Columbus, Ohio
Department of Cardiology
Cleveland Clinic
Cleveland, Ohio

Daniel J. Cantillon, MD
Co-chief Fellow
Cardiac Electrophysiology
Department of Cardiovascular
*   Medicine*
Cleveland Clinic
Cleveland, Ohio

Steven J. Filby, MD
Invasive Cardiology
Pinehurst Medical Center, Inc.
Pinehurst, North Carolina

Stephen Gimple, MD
Northland Cardiology
North Kansas City, Missouri

Brian W. Hardaway, MD
Staff, Heart Failure &
*   Transplantation*
HeartPlace at Baylor University
*   Medical Center*
Dallas, Texas

James E. Harvey, MD, MSc
Fellow of Cardiovascular Medicine
Heart and Vascular Institute
Cleveland Clinic
Cleveland, Ohio

Frederick A. Heupler, Jr, MD
Department of Cardiovascular Disease
Cleveland Clinic
Cleveland, Ohio

Robert E. Hobbs, MD
Kaufman Center for Heart Failure
Cleveland Clinic
Cleveland, Ohio

Arun Kalyanasundaram, MD, MPH
Interventional Cardiology Fellow
Cardiovascular Medicine
Cleveland Clinic
Cleveland, Ohio

Matthew Kaminski, MD
Cardiologist
Western Reserve Heart Care
University Hospitals Medical Practices
Assistant Professor of Medicine
Case Western Reserve University
    Cleveland, Ohio

A. Michael Lincoff, MD
Director, C5Research (Cleveland
    Clinic Coordinating Center
    for Clinical Research)
Director, Center for Clinical
    Research and Vice Chairman
    for Clinical Research, Lerner
    Research Institute
Vice Chairman, Department of
    Cardiovascular Medicine
Professor of Medicine, Cleveland
    Clinic Lerner College of
    Medicine of Case Western
    Reserve University
Cleveland Clinic
Cleveland, Ohio

Niranjan Seshadri, MD
Department of Cardiology
Harvard University Medical School
Beth Israel Deaconess Medical Center
Boston, Massachusetts

Mehdi H. Shishehbor, DO, MPH
Staff, Interventional Cardiology &
    Vascular Medicine
Cleveland Clinic
Cleveland, Ohio

Inder M. Singh, MD, MS
Interventional Cardiology Fellow
Division of Cardiovascular Diseases
Mayo Clinic
Rochester, Minnesota

Wilson H. Tang, MD
Department of Cardiovascular
    Medicine
Cleveland Clinic
Cleveland, Ohio

Preprocedural Evaluation

Bethany A. Austin

Cardiac catheterization is an invaluable tool for both diagnostic and therapeutic purposes, with between 2 and 3 million procedures performed annually in the United States. Due to the inherent risks associated with this invasive procedure, angiographers must be well versed in the indications, contraindications, and potential complications associated with this procedure. Thorough preprocedural evaluation facilitates appropriate selection of candidates for catheterization and identification of those at highest risk for complications.

Clinical Evaluation

Careful inquiry into a patient's clinical presentation is an essential component of the precatheterization evaluation. In addition to establishing the indication for catheterization, the clinical syndrome guides the selection of techniques employed during catheterization, including coronary angiography, hemodynamic measurements, left ventriculography, aortography, cerebral angiography, peripheral angiography, renal angiography, right heart catheterization, biopsy, and provocative chemical challenge.

Concomitant medical conditions should be identified and relevant comorbidities addressed prior to catheterization (Table 1-1). For example, severe thrombocytopenia or coagulopathy may render the patient ineligible for catheterization. In those with a prior history of heparin-induced thrombocytopenia, heparin-free solutions and flushes should be prepared. Alternate forms of anticoagulation, such as direct thrombin inhibitors, may be preferable for percutaneous intervention. In patients with chronic kidney disease (CKD), renal function should be optimized prior to catheterization (see Troubleshooting and Table 1-6).

Patients with severe lower extremity arterial disease may require catheterization via the brachial or radial artery. A history of an aortic aneurysm of significant size or prior aortic dissection may also favor

Table **1-1**	Relevant Historical Elements

A. Prior cardiac catheterizations and/or cardiac surgeries
B. Results of noninvasive cardiac imaging (echo, stress test, ECG)
C. Comorbid medical conditions
   1. Chronic kidney disease
   2. Diabetes mellitus
   3. Peripheral vascular disease
   4. Aortic aneurysm/dissection
   5. Valvular heart disease
   6. Thrombocytopenia/heparin-induced thrombocytopenia
   7. Coagulopathy
   8. Anemia
   9. Cerebrovascular disease
  10. Hypertension
  11. Pulmonary disease
  12. Liver disease
  13. Contrast allergy

brachial or radial artery access. Any history of claudication in conjunction with the peripheral pulse exam should be taken into account when selecting the arterial access site.

In patients with known pre-existing coronary artery disease, **detailed knowledge of all prior catheterizations, percutaneous interventions, and cardiac surgeries is imperative**. If possible, films of prior catheterizations should be reviewed for comparison. The angiographic location of prior bypass graft origins should be noted, as should any unusual catheters previously required. Knowledge of prior peripheral vascular interventions and surgeries is also useful in planning access.

Medication allergies should be documented prior to the procedure. In particular, patients with a history of contrast media allergy require special consideration (see Troubleshooting). Latex allergy is not a contraindication to cardiac catheterization; however, the catheterization laboratory should be notified of the allergy and be prepared to use only latex-free equipment for the case. Particular attention should also be paid to allergies to medications that are commonly used during the procedure, such as benzodiazepines and opiates.

A focused physical exam is a prerequisite for cardiac catheterization. Specifically, there should be an evaluation of any stigmata of congestive heart failure (CHF) such as rales, jugular venous distension, an S3, or peripheral edema. Auscultation of any murmurs, particularly those that suggest aortic stenosis or mitral regurgitation, should be noted. A careful examination of peripheral pulses and search for arterial bruits will influence the choice of arterial access site and serve as a helpful comparison when assessing for postprocedural vascular complications.

Standard laboratory evaluation includes **electrolytes, blood urea nitrogen, serum creatinine, blood glucose, and complete blood count. A coagulation panel is indicated in any patient on anticoagulant medication or who is at risk for significant hepatic dysfunction.** These laboratory tests should be current (i.e., within 1 month of the procedure). Similarly, a current electrocardiogram should be assessed. Evidence of ischemia, prior myocardial infarction (MI), rhythm disturbances, and chamber enlargement/hypertrophy should be noted. The baseline electrocardiogram also provides a comparison for any periprocedural changes. If a prior echocardiogram is available, preprocedural knowledge of left ventricular systolic or diastolic dysfunction, significant valvular disease, and aortic abnormalities is often helpful. Similarly, if a prior stress test is available, one should be familiar with areas of ischemia and scar.

Indications

The decision to proceed with diagnostic cardiac catheterization is based on a careful assessment of the risk–benefit ratio for the procedure (Table 1-2). The most current guidelines for diagnostic coronary angiography, reported by a joint Task Force of the American College of Cardiology and the American Heart Association (ACC/AHA), divide the indications for coronary angiography into three classes. Class I indications are conditions for which there is evidence and/or general agreement that the procedure is useful and effective. Class II indications are conditions for which there is conflicting evidence and/or a divergence of opinion about the usefulness/efficacy of performing the procedure. Class III indications are conditions for which there is evidence and/or general agreement that the procedure is not useful/effective and that in some cases may be harmful.

Cardiac catheterization is a powerful tool for risk stratification during acute MI and for facilitating revascularization. **Emergent coronary angiography with the intent to perform primary percutaneous coronary intervention is most applicable to patients presenting within 12 hours of an acute ST elevation or new left bundle branch block (LBBB) MI. This strategy can also be applied to patients with non–ST elevation MI who have persistent or recurrent symptoms despite optimal medical therapy or high-risk features which include elevated troponin,**

Table **1-2**	Indications for Coronary Angiography

Class I[ab]

Unstable Coronary Syndromes

    Unstable angina/ACS refractory to medical therapy or recurrent symptoms after initial medical therapy

    Unstable angina/ACS with high-risk indicators

    Unstable angina/ACS initially at low short-term risk, with subsequent high-risk noninvasive testing

    Prinzmetal angina with ST elevation

    Suspected acute or subacute stent thrombosis after PCI

Angina

    High-risk noninvasive testing

    CCS class III or IV angina on medical therapy

    Recurrent angina 9 months after PCI

Acute Myocardial Infarction

    Intended PCI in acute ST elevation or new LBBB MI

        Within 12 hours of symptom onset

        Ischemic symptoms persisting after 12 hours of symptom onset

        Cardiogenic shock in candidates for revascularization

        Persistent hemodynamic or electrical instability

    Angiography in non-ST elevation MI

        As part of an early invasive strategy in high-risk patients (+ troponin, ST changes, CHF, hemodynamic/electrical instability, recent revascularization)

        Persistent or recurrent symptomatic ischemia with or without associated ECG changes despite anti-ischemic therapy

        Resting ischemia or ischemia provoked by minimal exertion following infarction

    Prior to surgical repair of a mechanical complication of MI in a sufficiently stable patient

Perioperative Risk Stratification for Noncardiac Surgery

    High-risk noninvasive testing

    Unstable angina or angina unresponsive to medical therapy

    Equivocal noninvasive test result in patient with high clinical risk undergoing high-risk surgery

Congestive Heart Failure

    Systolic dysfunction associated with angina, regional wall motion abnormalities, or ischemia on noninvasive testing

Table **1-2**   (*Continued*)

Other Conditions

Valvular surgery in patients with angina, significant risk factor(s) for CAD, or abnormal noninvasive testing

Valvular surgery in men 35 or older, any postmenopausal woman, and premenopausal women 35 or older with cardiac risk factors

Correction of congenital heart disease in patients with angina, high-risk non-invasive testing, form of congenital heart disease frequently associated with coronary artery anomalies, or in those with known coronary anomalies

After successful resuscitation from sudden cardiac death, sustained monomorphic ventricular tachycardia, or nonsustained polymorphic ventricular tachycardia

Infective endocarditis with evidence of coronary embolization

Diseases of the aorta necessitating knowledge of concomitant coronary disease

Hypertrophic cardiomyopathy with angina

Class IIa[c]

Angina

CCS class I or II, EF <45%, and abnormal but not high-risk noninvasive testing

Patients with an uncertain diagnosis after noninvasive testing in whom the benefits of the procedure outweigh the risk

Patient who cannot be risk stratified by other means

Patients in whom nonatherosclerotic causes such as anomalous coronary artery, radiation vasculopathy, coronary dissection, etc. are suspected

Recurrent angina/symptomatic ischemia within 12 months of CABG

Recurrent angina poorly controlled with medical therapy after revascularization

Patients with CHF who have chest pain, have not had evaluation of their coronary anatomy, and do not have contraindications to revascularization

Acute Myocardial Infarction

MI suspected to have occurred by a mechanism other than thrombotic occlusion of atherosclerotic plaque (coronary embolism, arteritis, trauma, coronary spasm)

Failed thrombolysis with planned rescue PCI

Post MI with LVEF <40%, CHF, or malignant arrhythmias

CHF during acute episode with subsequent demonstration of LVEF >40%

Patients with recurrent ACS despite therapy without high-risk features

Perioperative Risk Stratification for Noncardiac Surgery

Planned vascular surgery with multiple intermediate clinical risk factors

Moderate-large region of ischemia on stress test without high-risk features or decreased EF

(*Continued on next page*)

Table **1-2**	*(Continued)*

Equivocal noninvasive testing in patient with intermediate clinical risk
undergoing high-risk surgery

Urgent noncardiac surgery while recovering from an acute MI

Other Conditions

Systolic LV dysfunction with unexplained cause after noninvasive testing

Episodic CHF with normal LV systolic function with suspicion for ischemia-
mediated LV dysfunction

Before corrective surgery for congenital heart disease in patients whose risk
factors increase likelihood of coronary disease

Recent blunt chest trauma and suspicion for acute MI

Before surgery for aortic dissection/aneurysm

Periodic follow-up after cardiac transplantation or for prospective immediate
cardiac transplant donors

Asymptomatic patients with Kawasaki disease and coronary artery aneurysms
on echocardiography

[a]ACC/AHA Guidelines adapted from Scanlon JP, Faxon DP, Audet AM, et al. ACC/AHA
guidelines for coronary angiography: executive summary and recommendations. A report of
the American College of Cardiology/American Heart Association Task Force on Practice
Guidelines (Committee on Coronary Angiography). *Circulation.* 1999;99:2345–2357; and Libby P,
Bonow RO, Mann DL, et al. *Braunwald's Heart Disease: A Textbook of Cardiovascular*
Medicine. 8th ed. Philadelphia: W.B. Saunders Company; 2007.
[b]Conditions for which there is evidence and/or general agreement that this procedure is
indicated.
[c]Conditions for which indications are controversial, but the weight of the evidence is
supportive.
ACS, acute coronary syndrome; CABG, coronary artery bypass graft, CAD, coronary artery disease, CCS, Canadian Cardiovascular Society, CHF, congestive heart failure, ECG, electrocardiogram, LBBB, left bundle branch block; LVEF, left ventricular ejection fraction, MI, myocardial
infarction, PCI, percutaneous coronary intervention.

**new ST depression, signs/symptoms of CHF, hemodynamic or elec-
trical instability, and prior revascularization.** Ideally, door-to-balloon
time in patients with ST elevation MI should be within 90 minutes.
Urgent angiography should also be performed in those patients younger
than 75 years with ST elevation MI complicated by cardiogenic shock developing within 36 hours of MI who are candidates for revascularization.
It is reasonable to include patient older than 75 years of age who have

good functional status and who are both suitable and agreeable to revascularization. Patients with persistent chest pain or ST elevation after fibrinolytic therapy should also have urgent angiography with the intent to perform primary percutaneous intervention. Additionally, patients who are successfully resuscitated from sudden cardiac death (without a readily identifiable cause) have a high probability of underlying coronary disease and should undergo cardiac catheterization.

During the hospital management phase following all types of MI, recurrent ischemia, malignant arrhythmias, clinical heart failure, and hemodynamic instability all warrant coronary angiography. Coronary angiography is indicated following all types of MI in patients with high-risk findings on stress testing, which include ST depression of ≥2 mm in multiple leads or persisting into recovery 6 minutes, ST elevation of ≥2 mm in leads without Q waves, a drop in blood pressure of 10 mm Hg or more with exercise, or development of ventricular tachycardia with stress. High-risk stress imaging findings include left ventricular dilatation, decrease in ejection fraction ≥10%, and multiple areas of ischemia.

An early invasive strategy with coronary angiography with the goal of revascularization should be utilized in patients presenting with unstable angina/non–ST elevation MI with high-risk indicators. This may be assessed using validated risk scoring systems such as the Thrombolysis in Myocardial Infarction (TIMI) or The Global Registry of Acute Coronary Events (GRACE) risk scores. Alternatively, clinical variables such as ST segment changes, positive troponin assays, signs/symptoms of CHF, new or worsening mitral regurgitation, decreased left ventricular systolic function <40%, and hemodynamic or electrical instability can be used. Additionally, patients with previous revascularization, particularly within the last 6 to 12 months, are considered at high risk. Any patient with UA/NSTEMI and a high-risk stress test result (see above) should proceed to coronary angiography. Depending on physician preference, patients with low-risk features may be further risk stratified with noninvasive testing prior to consideration of catheterization unless they develop recurrent severe or unstable angina despite medical management.

Development of ischemia after percutaneous coronary intervention may occur via acute or subacute stent thrombosis (<48 hours) or via instent restenosis (3–6 months). Similarly, surgical revascularization may be complicated by graft obstruction in the immediate perioperative period, or by graft disease that develops over time. **Suspected stent thrombosis warrants urgent catheterization and possible percutaneous coronary intervention.** Patients with recurrent angina or high-risk features on noninvasive testing within 9 months of successful percutaneous intervention or 12 months following coronary artery bypass graft surgery are

Table **1-3**	Canadian Cardiovascular Society Classification of Angina
Canadian Class	**Definition**
I	Ordinary physical activity does not cause angina
II	Slight limitation of ordinary activity (walking >2 blocks or climbing >1 flight of stairs)
III	Marked limitation of ordinary physical activity (walking 1–2 blocks or climbing 1 flight of stairs)
IV	Inability to carry on any activity without discomfort

also suitable candidates for coronary angiography. A low threshold for angiography is appropriate in patients with prior CABG in light of the variety of anatomic possibilities that can be provoking ischemia.

In patients with known or suspected coronary disease who are experiencing typical angina, the Canadian Cardiovascular Society classification of angina is a useful tool to gauge the severity of symptoms (Table 1-3). Patients with severe symptoms (CCS class III or IV) despite optimal medical therapy should undergo coronary angiography. Presence of high-risk criteria on noninvasive testing (see above) should also prompt coronary angiography in patients with known or suspected coronary disease, regardless of symptom severity. Patients with deterioration on serial noninvasive testing or patients with accelerating (crescendo) angina despite medical therapy should also be considered for angiography, even if noninvasive testing does not demonstrate high-risk features. **Routine angiography in asymptomatic patients without evidence of ischemia is not advocated.**

Atypical or nonspecific chest pain is infrequently due to myocardial ischemia. There are, however, several rare causes of ischemia that should be entertained in the differential diagnosis of atypical chest pain. These include Prinzmetal angina, cocaine abuse, coronary microvascular disease, pericarditis, myocarditis, coronary embolus, and aortic dissection. Noncardiac causes of chest pain include costochondritis, pleuritis, pulmonary embolus, and esophageal disorders. Due to the broad spectrum of possible etiologies for atypical chest pain, coronary angiography should be reserved for patients who demonstrate high-risk findings on noninvasive testing including ECG, or those in whom there is a clinical suspicion of coronary spasm meriting provocative testing.

The presence of left ventricular systolic dysfunction merits consideration of the possibility of concomitant coronary artery disease. Any patient with CHF in conjunction with reversible ischemia on noninvasive testing or regional wall motion abnormalities should be evaluated for coronary disease by angiography unless the patient is not a candidate for revascularization. Systolic dysfunction that is unexplained by noninvasive testing should also be further investigated by angiography.

In patients undergoing nonemergent surgery for valvular disease, coronary angiography is recommended for those at increased risk for concomitant coronary disease. Presence of chest pain, ischemia on noninvasive testing, decreased ejection fraction, or any significant risk factor for coronary disease all constitute class I indications for catheterization. Men 35 and older should have routine angiography prior to valvular surgery, as should postmenopausal women and premenopausal women 35 and older. In addition, patients with infective endocarditis who demonstrate evidence of coronary embolism should undergo coronary angiography. In patients with aortic valve endocarditis, particular care must be paid to catheter manipulation to avoid disrupting the vegetation, which could result in an embolic episode. Additionally, catheterization is indicated in those patients with symptomatic valvular lesions who have inconclusive or discordant noninvasive findings to obtain further diagnostic information such as hemodynamic measurements, transvalvular gradients, left ventricular pressure, aortography, or ventriculography.

In fact, when a cardiac surgical procedure is planned, patients with any significant risk factor(s) for coronary artery disease should undergo preoperative angiography, as should any with possible anginal symptoms. In preparing for surgical correction of congenital heart disease, those with chest pain or noninvasive testing suggestive of coronary artery disease should undergo diagnostic catheterization, as should those with conditions frequently associated with coronary anomalies that may complicate surgery. Patients in whom there is suspicion for malignant anomalies such as coronary artery stenosis, coronary arteriovenous fistula, and anomalous left coronary artery should also have diagnostic angiography prior to any correction. Additionally, patients with aortic disease such as dissection or aneurysm should have diagnostic catheterization prior to surgery or at any point in their clinical course when knowledge of the presence and extent of coronary artery disease is needed for management. In preparation for nonemergent, noncardiac surgery, those patients with evidence for high risk of adverse outcome based on noninvasive test results (i.e., suggestive of left main trunk [LMT] or multivessel disease), those with angina unresponsive to medical therapy and those with unstable angina should undergo coronary angiography prior to surgery.

It is equally important to be aware of conditions for which angiography is not indicated (Table 1-4). Patients who refuse, or who are ineligible for, revascularization should not undergo coronary angiography. **The only absolute contraindication to coronary angiography is the patient's refusal to undergo the procedure.** There are, however, several relative

Table **1-4**	Class III[a] Indications for Coronary Angiography[b]

Unstable Angina

Symptoms suggestive of unstable angina but without objective signs of ischemia and with a normal coronary angiogram during the past 5 years

Unstable angina in patients who are not revascularization candidates or for whom revascularization will not improve the quality or duration of life

Unstable angina in a post-bypass patient who is not a revascularization candidate

Patients with extensive comorbidities in whom risks of revascularization likely outweigh the benefits

Angina and Coronary Artery Disease

Angina in patients who do not desire revascularization

Screening test for CAD in asymptomatic patients

Patients with comorbidity in whom the risk outweighs the benefit of the procedure

Provocative testing in patients with high-grade obstructive disease

Nonspecific chest pain with normal noninvasive testing

Patients with CCS class I or II responsive to medical therapy with no ischemia on noninvasive testing

Routine angiography in asymptomatic patients after PCI or CABG (except in unprotected LMT PCI in which angiographic follow-up in 2–6 months is reasonable)

Myocardial Infarction: ST Segment Elevation or New LBBB

Patients beyond 12 hours from symptom onset who have no evidence of ongoing ischemia

After thrombolytic therapy with no evidence of ongoing ischemia

Routine angiography and PCI within 24 hours of thrombolytic therapy

Patients with extensive comorbidities in whom risks of revascularization likely outweigh benefits

All Myocardial Infarction: Hospital Management and Risk Stratification Phase

Patients who are not revascularization candidates or do not desire revascularization

Perioperative Risk Stratification for Noncardiac Surgery

Low-risk surgery with known CAD and no high-risk results on noninvasive testing

Asymptomatic after revascularization with excellent exercise capacity (>7 metabolic equivalents)

Table **1-4**	*(Continued)*

Mild stable angina, good left ventricular function, and not high risk by noninvasive testing

Patients who are not candidates for revascularization or do not desire revascularization

Part of work-up for renal, liver, or lung transplant without high-risk noninvasive test results

Valvular Heart Disease

Prior to surgery for infective endocarditis in patients lacking risk factors for CAD or evidence for coronary embolization

Routine angiography in patients not being assessed for surgery

[a]Conditions in which there is a consensus against the usefulness of the procedure.
[b]Adapted from Scanlon PJ, Faxon DP, Audet AM, et al. ACC/AHA guidelines for coronary angiography: executive summary and recommendations. A report of the American College of Cardiology/American Heart Association Task Force on Practice Guidelines (Committee on Coronary Angiography). *Circulation*. 1999;99:2345–2357; and Libby P, Bonow RO, Mann DL, et al. *Braunwald's Heart Disease: A Textbook of Cardiovascular Medicine*. 8th ed. Philadelphia: W.B. Saunders Company; 2007.
CAD, coronary artery disease; CCS, Canadian Cardiovascular Society; PCI, percutaneous coronary intervention; CABG, coronary artery bypass graft; LMT, left main trunk; LBBB, left bundle branch block.

contraindications (Table 1-5). These include a history of acute or advanced chronic renal failure, as contrast-induced or atheroembolic renal failure incurred during catheterization may significantly worsen pre-existing renal dysfunction. Gastrointestinal bleeding or unexplained anemia is a concern, especially if there is potential for percutaneous coronary intervention following diagnostic angiography, as this requires aggressive anticoagulation. Uncontrolled hypertension increases the risk of local vascular complications. Those patients with decompensated heart failure may not be able to tolerate lying flat and may suffer further deterioration from the contrast load.

Right heart, or pulmonary artery, catheterization can be performed simultaneously with left heart catheterization or in isolation depending on the clinical scenario. Indications for right heart catheterization include: acute MI associated with hemodynamic or mechanical complications, evaluation of etiology of shock and response to therapy, assessment of severity and potential reversibility of pulmonary hypertension, diagnosis of presence and significance of possible intracardiac shunt, and to delineate constrictive from restrictive physiology. For those patients with

Table **1-5**	Relative Contraindications to Coronary Angiography[a]

Acute renal failure or advanced chronic renal dysfunction
Active bleeding
Unexplained fever or significant leukocytosis
Untreated active infection
Acute stroke
Malignant hypertension
Significant electrolyte imbalance (i.e., K <3.0)
Patient unable to cooperate or does not desire revascularization
Concomitant severe illness reducing life expectancy
Digitalis toxicity
Decompensated heart failure or acute pulmonary edema precluding adequate
  patient positioning or oxygenation
Severe anemia or coagulopathy
Aortic valve endocarditis

[a]Adapted from Scanlon PJ, Faxon DP, Audet AM, et al. ACC/AHA guidelines for coronary angiography: a report of the American College of Cardiology/American Heart Association Task Force on Practice Guidelines (Committee on Coronary Angiography). *J Am Coll Cardiol.* 1999;33:1756–1824.

severe class IV CHF, right heart catheterization can be used both to diagnose the hemodynamic significance of their ventricular failure, to risk stratify them in the process of heart transplant evaluation, and to guide aggressive therapies such as ionotropic agent and intravenous afterload reduction. Additionally, right heart catheterization with endomyocardial biopsy is a routine component of the monitoring of post–heart transplant patients. Less compelling indications include assessment of volume status and diagnosis of cardiac tamponade. Right heart catheterization should not be performed in patients with right-sided thrombus or endocarditis or in those with mechanical tricuspid or pulmonic valve prostheses.

Angiography of the renal arteries remains the gold standard for evaluation of possible renal artery stenosis and should be considered in those patients with refractory hypertension, those with abrupt onset of hypertension, young patients with hypertension in whom fibromuscular dysplasia is a clinical consideration, or to confirm findings from a noninvasive study such as a renal Duplex ultrasound. An additional benefit of renal angiography is the ability to measure the gradients across any areas of stenosis. Similarly, cerebral angiography with digital subtraction angiography can be performed to definitively evaluate any cerebrovascular disease suspected clinically or, more typically, based on noninvasive findings. It allows visualization of the entire carotid circulation, including collateralization, and remains the gold standard. Additionally, cerebral angiography may be indicated in patients with infective endocarditis who require evaluation of possible mycotic aneurysm. However, the potential benefits must be weighed against the invasive nature of the test and possible neurologic complications, the incidence of which approaches 4%.

Angiography of the peripheral arteries can be performed to establish definitive diagnosis of peripheral arterial disease or subclavian stenosis. Indications include: preprocedural evaluation in those patients in whom revascularization is planned (class I), those who have significant symptoms from likely peripheral arterial disease such as rest pain or ulceration of the extremities, or for definitive diagnosis of peripheral arterial disease when noninvasive techniques are nondiagnostic.

Complications

The risk of major complications (death, MI, stroke) following diagnostic coronary angiography is generally less than 1%. However, several comorbid conditions significantly increase this baseline risk, including peripheral arterial disease, CKD, and diabetes mellitus requiring insulin therapy. Clearly, critically ill patients or those who have recently suffered a cardiac event are at higher risk than stable patients undergoing an elective procedure. Assessment of the patient's risk for complications is an important determinant of whether the procedure can be performed on an outpatient basis. Several factors favor short-term hospitalization after catheterization, including hydration for patients with chronic renal insufficiency and heparin bridging for mechanical prosthetic valves.

Obtaining informed consent for the catheterization is an integral part of preparing the patient. This discussion includes a thorough explanation of the indication for the procedure, the risks of administering conscious sedation, and the risks and benefits of the catheterization procedure. Although the risk of an adverse event for an individual patient does depend on the patient's comorbidities, the operator's experience, type of procedure, and the clinical setting in which the procedure is being performed, pooled frequencies of major complications may be used during an informed consent discussion.

The rate of death complicating coronary angiography has steadily fallen over the past 15 years and is now approximately 0.1%. High-risk features for periprocedural mortality include advanced age (age ≥60 years), advanced New York Heart Association functional class, severe left main coronary artery disease, and left ventricular systolic dysfunction (ejection fraction <30%). Baseline renal insufficiency, with worsening of renal function following catheterization, is associated with a particularly high mortality.

Periprocedural MI is fairly uncommon (≤0.1%). It is reasonable to check postprocedural cardiac enzymes in those at high risk. In the event of an ischemic complication during the procedure, it is advantageous to have cardiac surgical backup available. The patient and his or her family should be aware of the potential need for emergency coronary artery bypass surgery. Moreover, the patient and his or her family should be counseled about the potential need for percutaneous coronary intervention or coronary artery bypass graft surgery following the diagnostic procedure.

Periprocedural stroke rates have been quoted as ranging from 0.07% to 0.4%. Strokes are more common in patients with known cerebrovascular disease, hypertension, and severe aortic atherosclerosis. In such patients, catheter exchanges may be performed over a wire to minimize aortic atheromatous plaque disruption. Undoubtedly, patients with significant aortic stenosis who undergo retrograde valve catheterization are at increased risk for stroke. Patients who undergo catheterization following administration of thrombolytics or who receive high-dose anticoagulation, as well as those with advanced age or uncontrolled hypertension, are at increased risk for hemorrhagic stroke. The occurrence of periprocedural stroke has been associated with poor prognosis.

The incidence of vascular complication in diagnostic catheterization has fallen over the last decade with an incidence generally quoted as less than 1%. However, local vascular complications continue to be relatively common. Additionally, they are highly visible and distressing to the patient and are associated with significant morbidity. Local vascular complications are discussed in greater detail in Chapters 8 and 9.

Malignant arrhythmias such as ventricular tachycardia or ventricular fibrillation are rare. Minor ectopy and paroxysmal atrial arrhythmias are more common, but generally represent a benign and self-limited response to catheter manipulation. Bradycardia is the most common rhythm disturbance during catheterization, either in conjunction with a vasovagal reaction or in patients with pre-existing conduction disease. In particular, patients who have underlying LBBB who undergo right heart catheterization are at risk for advanced heart block.

The most common allergic reactions encountered during catheterization result from administration of contrast dye. Contrast dye allergies are relatively common, with up to 1% of patients developing some adverse reaction. Patients with known dye allergies should be premedicated with corticosteroids and antihistamines and should receive noniodinated contrast (see Troubleshooting and Table 1-6).

Renal dysfunction can result from administration of contrast agents, which is reported to occur in approximately 5% patients, or from renal

Troubleshooting

Precatheterization Preparation of Patients with Renal Dysfunction

Patients with any degree of renal impairment need to be well hydrated prior to cardiac catheterization, but it is essential in patients with a creatinine clearance <60 mL/min or a creatinine of >1.5. Hydration with 1 mL/kg/hr of either 0.9% or 0.45% saline for approximately 12 hours before and after the procedure has long been standard of care. In recent years, an alternative protocol using sodium bicarbonate 3 mL/kg for 1 hour prior to the procedure and 1 mL/kg for 6 hours after the procedure has also been shown to be at least as efficacious and is an appropriate hydration option as well. Modifications such as eliminating the bicarbonate bolus or decreasing the infusion rate or duration may be appropriate in patients who have a decreased left ventricular ejection fraction or a tenuous fluid balance.

Use of *N*-acetylcysteine (Mucomyst) 600 mg orally twice a day for four doses, two before the procedure and two afterward should also be considered. An increased dose of 1200 mg is reasonable in high-risk patients (creatinine >2.5 mg/dL or contrast load >140 mL). It is important to make patients with renal dysfunction who may require a coronary intervention aware of the possibility that a staged procedure may be a necessary precaution to minimize the contrast load.

Precatheterization Preparation of Patients with a Contrast Allergy

Patients with a documented contrast, iodine, or shellfish allergy should be premedicated with a regimen of corticosteroids (Prednisone 50–60 mg orally or Hydrocortisone 100 mg intravenously the night prior and the morning of the procedure) and antihistamines (Benadryl 25–50 mg orally or IV the night prior and the morning of the procedure) according to institutional preference (see Chapter 2 for more details).

atheroembolic disease, which is significantly less common. Renal atheroembolic disease complicates approximately 0.15% of cardiac catheterizations and should be suspected when acute renal failure occurs in conjunction with other clinical signs of embolization such as discolored toes, livedo reticularis, systemic or urinary eosinophilia, and abdominal pain.

While infection is generally not a common complication due to sterile technique, patients in whom a brachial approach is used and those in whom arterial closure devices are used are at a slightly higher risk. Toxic radiation exposure is also relatively uncommon, particularly in a straightforward diagnostic procedure where levels of exposure are often less than those received from a nuclear stress imaging study. However, special care should always be taken to minimize the amount of radiation exposure using the principle of "as low as reasonably achievable" without undue sacrifice of study quality. Additionally, those patients who have had recent radiation exposure in other catheterizations or procedures should receive additional counseling about the potential risk for toxicity including delayed skin burns.

Medication Considerations Prior to Coronary Angiography

In patients who are candidates for percutaneous coronary intervention after diagnostic angiography, aspirin 325 mg should be administered on the day of the procedure (Table 1-6). The use of clopidogrel (600 mg loading dose) prior to catheterization may be indicated in patients who are likely to undergo percutaneous coronary intervention. This must be weighed against the possibility that they will require coronary artery bypass graft surgery, which often must be postponed for several days after administration of clopidogrel. **Warfarin should be stopped several days before the procedure. Ideally, the international normalized ratio**

Table **1-6**	Preprocedural Medication Considerations
Medication	**Adjustment**
Aspirin	325 mg orally prior to the procedure
Clopidogrel	600 mg oral loading dose if there is a high probability of PCI
Glycoprotein IIb–IIIa Inhibitor	Continue if already started; may be started on arrival to lab if PCI planned
Unfractionated heparin	Per discretion of operator, but generally held on patient transport to catheterization lab
Low molecular weight heparin	Per discretion of operator
Warfarin	Hold for 2–3 days prior to procedure until INR <1.5–1.8; heparin or low molecular weight heparin can be used if continued anticoagulation is essential
Insulin and hypoglycemics	Hold on the morning of the procedure
Metformin	Hold on the day prior to procedure and resume 2 days after procedure if renal function remains unchanged
Acetylcysteine (Mucomyst)	600–1200 mg orally twice daily starting the day prior to the procedure for patients with chronic renal dysfunction

PCI, percutaneous coronary intervention.

should be less than 1.5 to 1.8 prior to catheterization, depending on operator comfort and acuity of the indication. Heparin (3,000 to 5,000 units IV) should be considered for patients undergoing cardiac catheterization via an arm approach.

Metformin is eliminated primarily via the kidneys and therefore accumulates among patients with renal insufficiency (glomerular filtration rate <70 mL/min, or serum creatinine >1.6 mg/dL). Contrast media can impair renal function and lead to further retention of metformin, which is known to precipitate the onset of lactic acidosis. The incidence of lactic acidosis associated with metformin, regardless of exposure to contrast media, is 0.03 cases per 1,000 patients per year, and 50% result in death. There is no conclusive evidence to indicate that contrast media precipitates the development of metformin-induced lactic acidosis among patients with normal serum creatinine (<1.5 mg/dL). This complication is almost exclusively observed among non–insulin dependent diabetic patients with abnormal renal function before injection of contrast media. **Metformin should be held the day prior to the procedure and restarted 2 days after the procedure if renal function remains unchanged.**

Long-acting oral hypoglycemics and insulin should be held 12 to 24 hours prior to the procedure depending on their duration of action. In general, diuretics should be held 12 to 24 hours prior to the procedure in an effort to avoid excessive nephrotoxicity unless of course the patient's volume status is tenuous.

General Suggested Reading

Baim DS, Grossman W, eds. *Cardiac Catheterization, Angiography, and Intervention*. 7th ed. Philadelphia: Lippincott Williams and Wilkins; 2006.

Kern MJ. *The Cardiac Catheterization Handbook*. 4th ed. St. Louis: Mosby-Year Book; 2003.

Libby P, Bonow RO, Mann DL, et al., eds. *Braunwald's Heart Disease: A Textbook of Cardiovascular Medicine*. 8th ed. Philadelphia: W.B. Saunders Company; 2007.

Topol EJ, ed. *Textbook of Interventional Cardiology*. 5th ed. Philadelphia: Saunders/Elsevier; 2008.

Chapter 1 Suggested Reading

Ashley KE, Cho L. Right heart catheterization. In: Griffin BP, Topol EJ, eds. *Manual of Cardiovascular Medicine*. 3rd ed. Philadelphia: Lippincott Williams and Wilkins; 2009:743–756.

Anwarrudin S. Left heart catheterization. In: Griffin BP, Topol EJ, eds. *Manual of Cardiovascular Medicine*. 3rd ed. Philadelphia: Lippincott Williams and Wilkins; 2009:789–813.

Carrozza JP. Complications of diagnostic cardiac catheterization. *UpToDate.* 2008;Version 16.3.

Davidson CJ, Bonow RO. Cardiac catheterization. In: Libby P, Bonow RO, Mann DL, et al., eds. *Braunwald's Heart Disease: A Textbook of Cardiovascular Medicine.* 8th ed. Philadelphia: W.B. Saunders Company; 2007:439–464.

Heupler FA, Proudfit WL, Razavi M, et al. Ergonovine maleate provocative test for coronary arterial spasm. *Am J Cardiol.* 1978;41:631–640.

Laskey W, Boyle J, Johnson LW. Multivariable model for prediction of risk of significant complication during diagnostic cardiac catheterization: the Registry Committee of the Society for Cardiac Angiography and Interventions. *Cathet Cardiovasc Diagn.* 1993;30:185–190.

Maeder M, Klein M, Fehr T, et al. Contrast nephropathy: review focusing on prevention. *J Am Coll Cardiol.* 2004;44:1763–1771.

Mueller HS, Chatterjee K, Davis KB, et al. ACC Expert Consensus Document: Present use of Bedside Right Heart Catheterization in patients with cardiac disease. *J Am Coll Cardiol.* 1998;32:840–864.

Ryan TJ, Anderson JL, Antman EM, et al. ACC/AHA guidelines for the management of patients with acute myocardial infarction: a report of the American College of Cardiology/American Heart Association Task Force on Practice Guidelines (Committee on the Management of Acute Myocardial Infarction). *J Am Coll Cardiol.* 1996;28:1328–1428.

Antman EM, Hand M, Armstrong PW, et al. 2007 Focused Update of the ACC/AHA 2004 Guidelines for the Management of Patients with ST-Elevation Myocardial Infarction. A Report of the American College of Cardiology/American Heart Association Task Force on Practice Guidelines. *Circulation.* 2008;117:1–34.

Scanlon PJ, Faxon DP, Audet AM, et al. ACC/AHA guidelines for coronary angiography: executive summary and recommendations. A report of the American College of Cardiology/American Heart Association Task Force on Practice Guidelines (Committee on Coronary Angiography). *Circulation.* 1999;99:2345–2357.

Scanlon PJ, Faxon DP, Audet AM, et al. ACC/AHA guidelines for coronary angiography: a report of the American College of Cardiology/American Heart Association Task Force on Practice Guidelines (Committee on Coronary Angiography). *J Am Coll Cardiol.* 1999;33:1756–1824.

Wilterdink JL, Furie KL, Kistler JP. Evaluation of carotid artery stenosis. *UpToDate.* 2008;Version 16.3.

CHAPTER 2

Setting up the Lab

Matthew Kaminski

Prior to arrival of the patient, the catheterization team should verify that all monitoring, recording, and resuscitation equipment are functioning properly. Continuous monitoring of the patient's ECG upon arrival to the catheterization laboratory is indispensable since it can quickly identify any arrhythmias, conduction abnormalities, or evidence of ischemia. An automated blood pressure cuff and continuous pulse oximetry are also necessary. Resuscitation equipment such as intubation trays and defibrillators should be tested and placed nearby. If a patient is unable to urinate lying flat or if a long cardiac catheterization is expected, a Foley or Texas urinary catheter should be placed.

Time-Out Protocol

The concept of preprocedural verification using a verbal "time-out" was originally developed as a patient-safety measure to prevent wrong-site surgery; however, it has evolved to become standard protocol before any medical procedure and should be performed before every procedure in the cardiac catheterization lab. The purpose of the time-out immediately before starting the procedure is to conduct a final assessment that the correct patient, site, positioning, and procedure are identified and that all relevant documents, related information, and necessary equipment are available. Each catheterization lab should have a standardized time-out protocol. The time-out should be performed prior to the introduction of local anesthesia and sedation, should be initiated by a physician operator, and all staff participating in the case (nurses, technicians, etc.) should be involved. It should involve interactive verbal communication between all team members, and any team member should be able to express concerns about the procedure verification. During the time-out, other activities are suspended, to the extent possible without compromising patient safety, so that all relevant members of the team are focused on the active confirmation of the correct patient, procedure, site, and other critical elements. All time-outs should address the topics listed in Table 2-1.

Table **2-1**	Essential Elements of a Preprocedural Time-Out

Patient identification (name and medical record number)
Confirmation of correct site marking (for percutaneous access)
Accuracy of preprocedure consent documentation
Correct patient positioning
Specification of procedure to be performed
Safety precautions based on patient history or medication use (allergies)
Special (nonroutine) equipment or instruments required

Preprocedural Sedation: In nonemergent situations, a detailed discussion with the patient and family explaining the cardiac catheterization procedure, potential complications, and alternative diagnostic options helps to alleviate any anxiety prior to the procedure. Prior to administration of preprocedural sedation, the operator should ascertain that informed consent has been obtained and that all of the patient's questions have been answered.

The objective of preprocedural sedation is to maximize procedure safety by making the patient cooperative, calm, and relaxed. The goal should be to achieve **conscious sedation: a state where the patient has a depressed level of consciousness but still maintains the independent ability to preserve a patent airway and respond appropriately and quickly to verbal and/or physical stimuli.** Prior to administration of preprocedural sedation, the operator should examine the patient with special attention to the airway to identify patients who may require additional caution with the use of sedative agents (e.g., sleep apnea, laryngeal mass, intrinsic pulmonary disease).

Factors that may influence the selection and dose of sedative include the patient's age and weight, anticipated procedure length, comorbid medical illnesses, level of anxiety, pain threshold, drug allergies, and potential drug interactions. If preprocedural sedation is initiated with oral medications, they should be administered at least 1 hour prior to the patient arriving at the catheterization laboratory. Table 2-2 lists commonly used medications for preprocedural sedation and their antagonists. A benzodiazepine is usually the initial drug of choice since it is not only a sedative and anxiolytic, but also achieves a limited degree of retrograde amnesia. Midazolam (Versed) is often the preferred choice because of its rapid onset of action and relative short duration of effect. Initial doses range from 0.5 to 1 mg IV, which may be repeated every few minutes until desired sedation is achieved. If further sedation is needed, administering a

Table **2-2**	Commonly Used Doses of Preprocedural Sedation Medications		
Medication	**Oral Dose**	**IV Dose**	**Comments**
Benzodiazepines			
Diazepam (Valium)	5–10 mg	2–5 mg	
Lorazepam (Ativan)	0.5–2 mg	1–2 mg	
Midazolam (Versed)	N/A	0.5–2 mg	
Opioids			
Fentanyl	N/A	25–50 μg	
Morphine sulfate	15–30 mg	1–4 mg	
Meperidine (Demerol)	50–150 mg	50–100 mg	
Antihistamines			
Diphenhydramine (Benadryl)	25–50 mg	25–50 mg	
Promethazine (Phenergan)	25–50 mg	12.5–25 mg	
Antagonists			
Naloxone (Narcan)	N/A	0.4–2 mg	Opioid overdose: repeat dose every 2–3 minutes to achieve effect or to a maximum dose of 10 mg
Flumazenil (Romazicon)	N/A	0.2–0.5 mg	Benzodiazepine overdose: repeat dose every minute to achieve effect or to a maximum dose of 3 mg

short-acting opioid such as fentanyl (25–50 μg) often results in adequate patient comfort.

Contrast Agents

Overview of Available Contrast Agents: Iodinated contrast media are the most frequently used intravascular pharmacologic agents in the world. More than 70 million injections are administered worldwide

Table **2-3**	Contrast Agents				
Class	**Generic Name**	**Trade Name**	**Iodine**	**Osmolality**	**Viscosity**
Low osmolar	Iohexol	Omnipaque	350	844	10.4
	Iopamidol	Isovue 370	370	796	9.4
	Ioversol	Optiray 320	320	702	5.8
	Ioxilan	Oxilan 350	350	695	8.1
Iso-osmolar	Iodixanol	Visipaque 320	320	290	11.8

Iodine (mg/mL), osmolality (mOsm/kg H_2O), viscosity (37 F).

each year. All intravascular contrast agents contain iodine, which absorbs x-rays to a greater degree than surrounding tissue and allows for intravascular opacification. Iodine atoms are bound to carbon-based molecules, making the agent water soluble. Contrast agents are classified based on their osmolality (high, low, or iso-osmolal). High-osmolar contrast media (HOCM) were the first intravascular contrast agents developed in the 1950s. They have an osmolality five to eight times greater than that of plasma (approximately 2,000 mOsm/kg). In the 1980s, low osmolar contrast media (LOCM) were created, having an osmolality of two to three times that of plasma (600–800 mOsm/kg). Then, in the 1990s, the first iso-osmolar contrast media (IOCM), iodixanol, was developed, with an osmolality of 290 mOsm/kg. Given the substantially higher rates of adverse effects with use of HOCM, these agents are effectively obsolete and are no longer used clinically. Thus, all currently available contrast media are either LOCM or IOCM. Table 2-3 lists examples of the commonly used contrast agents used in coronary angiography.

Adverse Effects: Many of the studies that have attempted to differentiate the various adverse effects of specific LOCM have been contradictory, making it difficult to make firm recommendations for use of a particular agent. Selection of a particular LOCM varies among institutions and operators and is often made based on personal experience and preference. Some basic guidelines regarding the choice of agent will be presented in the following sections.

Effect on Myocardial Function: The degree of myocardial depression, peripheral vasodilation, and elevation of left ventricular filling pressures seen with contrast agents is more marked with agents that have higher osmolality. This is even more apparent when larger boluses of contrast agents are used during ventriculography or aortography. When HOCM were used routinely, it was not uncommon to have peripheral vasodilation with a transient reduction in systolic blood pressure of 20 to 50 mm Hg and corresponding compensatory increase in heart rate with the use of high osmotic agents. **These hemodynamic perturbations could be particularly catastrophic in patients with relatively low cardiac reserve such as left main coronary artery disease, severe aortic stenosis, or severe left ventricular dysfunction (see Chapter 7).** In contrast, the LOCM used today typically only cause a reduction in systolic blood pressure of 5 to 15 mm Hg with no change in heart rate during ventriculography or aortography. Despite the more minor hemodynamic effects, caution must still be used when performing these procedures in potentially unstable patients.

Electrophysiologic Effects: Injection of contrast media into the coronary arteries can rarely cause ventricular fibrillation or sinus bradycardia, occasionally leading to transient sinus arrest. The incidence of these events is low. Series with nonionic LOCM found an incidence of 0.1% for ventricular fibrillation and 0.2% for bradycardia.

Effect on Renal Function: Contrast-induced acute kidney injury (AKI) is the most common and most serious adverse effect of intravascular contrast administration. Contrast-induced AKI is typically defined as an increase in serum creatinine of at least 0.5 mg/dL or 25% increase above baseline that occurs within the first 24 hours after contrast administration and peaks within the first 5 days. It is estimated that approximately 7% of patients receiving intravascular contrast will suffer AKI. It has been shown that these patients have up to a fivefold increase in the risk of in-hospital death over matched controls who did not develop contrast-induced AKI. Overall, less than 1% of patients who suffer contrast-induced nephropathy ultimately require chronic dialysis. Various factors (Table 2-4) may predispose a patient to deterioration in renal function after the use of contrast agents. Of these, chronic kidney disease (CKD) with reduction in estimated glomerular filtration rate (GFR)

Table **2-4**   **Risk Factors for Contrast-induced Nephropathy**
Estimated GFR <60 mL/min/m^2
Diabetes mellitus
Hypovolemia
Hypotension or shock
High contrast volumes (greater than 3 mL/kg)

below 60 mL/min/m^2 is the most significant. Patients with CKD have a reduced number of nephrons. The remaining healthy nephrons are susceptible to damage by iodinated contrast, leading to contrast-induced AKI. After intravascular administration of contrast material, the kidney responds by releasing potent renal vasoconstrictors, which reduce renal blood flow by up to 50%. The reduced blood flow leads to concentration of contrast in the renal tubules and collecting ducts, which allows for direct cellular injury and death to renal tubular cells. The degree of toxicity to tubular cells is related to the length of time the cells are exposed to contrast, highlighting the importance of high urinary flow rates before contrast administration.

Prevention of Contrast-induced AKI: There are several strategies to reduce the risk of contrast-induced AKI in susceptible patients. Prior to contrast administration, potentially nephrotoxic drugs such as non-steroidal anti-inflammatory drugs (NSAIDs), calcineurin inhibitors, high-dose loop diuretics, and aminoglycosides should be held for several days, if possible. In addition, volume expansion and treatment of dehydration have been shown to prevent AKI in clinical studies. There is limited data to recommend an optimal prehydration strategy, but it appears that isotonic crystalloid such as normal saline or sodium bicarbonate are more effective than half-normal saline. Despite some recent enthusiasm that isotonic bicarbonate may be superior to normal saline in the prevention of contrast-induced AKI, the largest clinical trial to date showed no clear advantage for bicarbonate over saline. There is also little data on the optimum urinary flow rate. One study found that urinary flow rate of >150 mL/hr in the 6 hours after the procedure was associated with reduced rates of AKI. To obtain this, however, isotonic crystalloid needs to be administered at 1.0 to 1.5 mL/kg/min, owing to the loss of some fluid to the interstitial space.

There are currently no approved pharmacologic agents to prevent contrast-induced AKI. Despite its popularity, *N*-acetylcysteine (NAC) has not been consistently shown to be effective in preventing AKI. The only treatment that has been shown to be effective is high-dose ascorbic acid. The dose used in the one prospective trial published was 3 g orally the night before contrast exposure and 2 g orally twice a day for 1 day after the procedure.

Once contrast is administered, **limiting contrast volume for all patients to less than 5 mL/kg divided by the serum creatinine has been shown to be associated with lower rates of contrast-induced AKI. For patients with CKD, use of as little contrast as possible (<30 mL if possible) appears to be related to a reduction in subsequent dialysis.** It should be noted, however, that even small volumes of contrast can have adverse effects on renal function in patients at high risk for AKI. For these patients, there is no safe dosing threshold below which there is no risk of AKI. It is recommended that contrast volumes below 100 mL are preferable in patients who have an estimated GFR <60 mL/min/m².

The choice of contrast agent is also a major factor in determining the risk of contrast-induced AKI. Use of LOCM confers a significantly lower risk of AKI compared to HOCM. However, multiple trials have shown that IOCM has the lowest risk for contrast-induced AKI, especially in patients with CKD and diabetes mellitus (DM). Currently, iodixanol (Visipaque, GE Healthcare Biosciences/Amersham Health, Piscataway, NJ) is the only clinically available IOCM. An expert panel has recommended that in patients undergoing angiographic procedures with CKD with estimated glomerular filtration rate (eGFR) <60 mL/min/m², and particularly those with DM, iodixanol presents the lowest risk of contrast-induced AKI and should be the contrast agent of choice. It is also recommended that iodixanol be used in renal dialysis patients to minimize the chances of volume overload and associated complications before the next dialysis session.

Contrast Reactions: Adverse reactions to contrast media are not uncommon. Mild adverse reactions are reported in 3% to 12% of patients receiving contrast, with mortality rates of less than 1 in 100,000. Reactions are much more frequent with ionic contrast media, which are no longer in use in the majority of centers. Adverse reactions are typically classified as either immediate (occurring within 1 hour of administration) or delayed (between 1 hour and 1 week later). Immediate reactions can range from mild to very severe with symptoms of nausea, pruritus, urticaria and angioedema, to bronchospasm, laryngeal edema, hypotension, and even death. They account for approximately a quarter of all contrast reactions. Delayed reactions are usually mild to moderate skin reactions, which become apparent between 3 hours and 3 days after exposure and resolve without treatment within 1 week. Table 2-5 outlines common presentation and treatment of immediate contrast reactions. A great deal of controversy exists regarding the exact mechanism of contrast reactions, but it is thought that **the majority of reactions are not mediated by immunoglobin E, and thus are not truly allergic**. Multiple investigators have demonstrated conclusively, however, that immediate reactions involve the granular release of histamine by mast cells and basophils, producing an anaphylactoid response. Regardless of the mechanism, the risk of a reaction to contrast is increased twofold in patients with a strong history of allergy or atopy such as asthma. A common misconception is that a prior reaction to seafood confers a greatly elevated risk of an adverse reaction with contrast exposure. In reality, patients with allergies to seafood have a similar risk of contrast reactions as those who have a strong history of other allergic reactions. Patients with

Table 2-5 Contrast Reactions: Presentation and Treatment

Severity	Presentation	Onset	Treatment
Mild	Mild nausea, flushing, bradycardia, urticaria without hives or tongue swelling, transient bradycardia or vasovagal episodes	Within minutes of exposure	Usually self-limited; supportive treatment usually includes observation and/or diphenhydramine 25–50 mg PO; atropine (0.5–1.0 mg IV) occasionally required
Moderate	Persistent nausea with vomiting, anaphylactoid reaction (urticaria with hives and tongue swelling), persistent symptomatic bradycardia or vasovagal episodes	Within minutes to hours of exposure	Usually requires treatment consisting of IV hydration, antihistamines (diphenhydramine 50 mg IV and famotidine 20 mg IV), steroids (i.e., hydrocortisone 100 mg IV), antiemetics (i.e., prochlorperazine 2 mg IV), and atropine (0.5–2.0 mg IV) if persistent bradycardia and/or vasovagal reaction; epinephrine (0.1–0.3 mL of 1:1,000 concentration) SQ or IM to treat bronchspasm without hypotension
Severe	Anaphylaxis-like (bronchospasm, laryngeal edema, and hypotension)	Can occur immediately after a single dose of contrast	Life threatening and requires immediate and aggressive treatment; epinephrine (1 mL of 1:10,000 solution) (0.1 mg/ml) IV q 1 min PRN, steroids (i.e., hydrocortisone 100 mg IV), antihistamines (diphenhydramine 50 mg IV and famotidine 20 mg IV), and rapid IV fluid expansion; consider intubation if airway compromised

Troubleshooting

Managing patients with a history of prior contrast reactions: Patients with a prior moderate or severe reaction to contrast agents should be premedicated with steroids and antihistamines prior to contrast exposure. Protocols vary widely, but commonly used regimens include 50 mg of oral prednisone 13, 7, and 1 hour prior to the procedure (q6 hours) along with diphenhydramine 50 mg IV or PO 1 hour prior to the procedure. Intravenous steroids can be substituted for oral steroids with hydrocortisone 200 mg IV 1 hour prior to contrast administration.

a previous adverse reaction to contrast have about a sixfold increased risk of an adverse reaction upon repeat exposure to contrast when compared with individuals without a prior adverse reaction. This elevated risk justifies pharmacologic prophylaxis with steroids and histamine blockade prior to planned repeat contrast exposure for patients with a history of moderate or severe reactions, although it should be noted that data is very limited on the efficacy of these preventive pharmacologic measures when modern-day nonionic LOCM or IOCM is used. Physicians should also note that serious, life-threatening reactions have been reported despite the use of steroid and antihistamine prophylaxis!

Radiation Safety

The main principle regarding radiation safety in cardiology is to keep exposure to the patient and operator to a level as low as reasonably achievable (ALARA). The principle of ALARA is achieved by learning the various techniques at reducing radiation exposure and their possible effects on image quality (Table 2-6). If these techniques are not learned, radiation exposure to the operator and/or patient may result in direct tissue injury (deterministic effects) and/or neoplasms and heritable alterations in reproductive cells (stochastic effects).

Operators should wear radiation dosimeter badges whenever they are working with a source of radiation. They should be worn at collar level either on the apron or attached to the thyroid shield. These badges are monitored at periodic intervals (usually monthly). **The annual total effective whole-body dose limit for occupational radiation workers is 5 rem/year (50 mGy/year).**

The main source of radiation exposure for the operator is scatter from the patient. A secondary, less significant, source is escape of x-rays through the shielding of the x-ray tube. Protection for the operator consists of shielding, proper positioning from the radiation source,

Table **2-6**	Radiation Safety Principles and Corresponding Effects on Image Quality		
Method	Operator Dose	Patient Dose	Image Quality
Patient and Operator Protection			
Lead gown, thyroid collar	Reduced	Unchanged	Unchanged
Leaded glasses	Reduced	Unchanged	Unchanged
Lead shield above, below table	Reduced	Unchanged	Unchanged
Increased distance from operator to table	Reduced	Unchanged	Unchanged
Femoral vs. brachial approach	Reduced	Unchanged	Unchanged
Operator's fingers out of radiation beam	Reduced	Unchanged	Unchanged
Move patient's arm out of field	Reduced	Reduced	Improved
Radiation Dose Reduction			
Shorter fluoroscopy, cine times	Reduced	Reduced	Unchanged
Pulsed fluoroscopy	Reduced	Reduced	Unchanged
Fewer pulses per second	Reduced	Reduced	Worse
Fewer cine frames per second	Reduced	Reduced	Worse
Greater distance from source to patient	Variable	Reduced	Improved
Shorter distance from image intensifier to patient	Reduced	Reduced	Improved
Electronic image magnification	Variable	Higher	Improved
Smaller collimator opening	Variable	Variable	Improved
Cranial, caudal angulation	Higher	Higher	Worse
Large patient, pleural effusion	Higher	Higher	Worse

and adjusting the fluoroscopic controls in an attempt to minimize radiation exposure while maintaining a high-quality image.

Personal shielding involves lead aprons, thyroid collars, and lead glasses. **Lead aprons should have shielding properties equivalent to 0.5 mm of lead, which shields the covered areas of the operator from roughly 90% of scatter radiation.** Lead glasses protect the operator from possible radiation-induced cataracts and should have side shields to decrease radiation from the lateral direction. Thyroid shields prevent large cumulative doses of radiation that could lead to thyroid cancer. These items should be checked annually with fluoroscopy to inspect for possible cracks, holes, and other signs of deterioration. The catheterization table will commonly have two lead shields: one which is a table side drape that protects the lower body of the operator, and one that is an adjustable lead acrylic shield which is suspended from the ceiling to aid in the protection of the operator's head and upper torso.

The inverse square law addresses the important concept that radiation dose drops rapidly by the inverse square of the relative increase of distance from the radiation source. Operators can decrease their radiation exposure by taking a step back from the irradiated area before engaging in fluoroscopy. Moving the image intensifier, which is located above the patient, to as close to the patient as possible also reduces scatter radiation by reducing geometric magnification (radiation dose usually increases with the square of the magnification). Placing hands in the direct beam of radiation should only be done in cases of emergency.

Modifying fluoroscopic controls can also decrease radiation exposure for both the operator and the patient; however, these modifications may occasionally reduce image quality. One of the "golden rules" for minimizing radiation exposure is **keeping beam-on time to an absolute minimum.** Fluoroscopy or cineangiography should not be engaged if the image on the monitor is not being used. Most fluoroscopic machines have an option that allows the operator to select the level of image quality (low, normal, high). Low image quality reduces radiation dose rate, but often produces a noisy image. These images may be acceptable in certain situations such as checking position of a guidewire or catheter. Most fluoroscopic machines have pulsed fluoroscopy which results in x-rays being produced in short bursts instead of a continuous stream as in conventional fluoroscopy. Reducing the pulse frequency to 15 or 7.5 pulses of x-rays/second will reduce radiation exposure at the cost of producing a somewhat flickering, choppy image. A similar result is seen when one reduces the cine frame rate. Applying collimators (blades outside the x-ray tube that block x-rays) to the area of interest not only reduces scatter radiation to the operator, but also improves image quality.

Electronic magnification (field-of-view) size for image intensifiers consists of usually at least three magnifications: 9-in (23-cm), 7-in (17-cm), and 5-in (13-cm). In general, the least magnification reduces the dose rate to the patient's skin. For example, without changing collimators, changing the field of view from 7 to 5-in results in roughly a doubling in entrance dose to the patient's skin, with greater spatial resolution that may be important in evaluating small coronary arteries. The effect of increasing magnification on radiation dose rates for the operator and other personal is variable since it depends on the relative changes in tube current and kilovoltage.

Increasing the distance between the x-ray source (located beneath the patient) and the patient also results in improved image quality and a reduction in entry dose to the skin of the patient. Federal regulations dictate that a spacer be placed on the x-ray tube to maintain a minimum distance of 38 cm between the x-ray source and the patient.

Needle, Catheter, Wire, Sheath Selection

Access Needle: Access needles typically consist of two types, an open-bore needle and a Seldinger-type needle, which has a stylet in place. Open-bore needles are easier to manage since they signal immediate blood return when the vessel of interest is punctured. However, they may have to be flushed periodically if repeated attempts at access are needed because they can become clogged with subcutaneous tissue, fat, or blood. The stylet in the Seldinger-type needle prevents blockage of the lumen of the needle with tissue or blood and is removed once the operator believes puncture of the artery has occurred.

Most needles have a standard length of between 2.75 and 3 in. A 1.5-in 21-gauge or 22-gauge needle is commonly used for the percutaneous radial approach. Needles are conventionally sized by their outer diameter, which corresponds to an arbitrary gauging system. Increasing gauge corresponds to a smaller diameter. Typically, an 18-gauge needle is used for the femoral or brachial approach, while a micropuncture kit containing a 22-gauge needle is used for the radial approach. When attempting access for left heart catheterization, the needle should be held at its hub so that the operator can feel arterial pulsations transmitted from the tip of the needle. Feeling these pulsations aids in guiding the operator to successful cannulation of the arterial circulation.

Guidewire: Once access is obtained, a guidewire is inserted into the needle prior to withdrawal of the needle and placement of an arterial sheath over the guidewire. Guidewires are also used to facilitate passage of diagnostic coronary catheters to the central aorta. The choice of guidewire should be made prior to obtaining arterial access. Most guidewires consist of three major components: a central core (commonly stainless steel or nitinol), distal flexible spring coil (usually platinum or tungsten), and an outer coating to decrease friction (silicone, Teflon, or other hydrophilic coating). If a patient has severely tortuous or atherosclerotic vessels, a flexible wire such as a Wholey wire can be used. Alternatively, a Glidewire (SCIMED) may be of particular benefit because it has smooth hydrophilic coating and excellent torque control. Guidewire length varies among different manufacturers, but generally consists of three major types. Short wires (30–45 cm) are used in placing sheaths. Medium length wires (125–150 cm) enable the operator to guide the diagnostic coronary catheter to the aorta. Long length wires (250–300 cm) are employed when the operator wishes to exchange diagnostic coronary catheters without moving the wire tip ("exchange wire"). Wire tips are universally flexible and are either straight or J-tipped. **For the majority of cases, the J-tipped wire is preferred since it is less likely to induce vessel dissection and avoids entering small vessel branches.** A straight-tipped wire is used mainly in attempting to cross a severely stenotic aortic valve or in obtaining brachial or radial arterial access.

Guidewire diameters also vary widely. The smaller diameter guidewires (0.018, 0.021, and 0.025 in) are generally used with a Swan–Ganz catheter to augment stiffness. The 0.025-in guidewire is also used in obtaining radial arterial access. The 0.032-in guidewire is used mostly in brachial arterial access and intra-aortic balloon placement. The most commonly used guidewires are the 0.035 and 0.038-in, used during most routine diagnostic left heart catheterizations. The 0.035-in wire is usually preferred because it is more flexible and softer, thus less likely to cause a dissection. The 0.038-in wire is used when increased stiffness is desired, such as when attempting dilator placement through calcified arteries or fibrotic tissue. Larger diameter guidewires are used predominantly in interventional cases where larger sheaths and catheter sizes are often necessary.

Dilators and Sheaths: Vascular sheaths generally contain a removable dilator, a diaphragm that prevents leakage of blood or air into the sheath, and a side arm that is connected to a three-way stopcock that allows the operator to record pressure measurements, flush the sheath, and infuse medications. The dilator is made of stiff plastic (usually Teflon or polyethylene) that allows it to pass through fibrous subcutaneous tissue or atherosclerotic/calcified vessels. Generally, the sheaths used range from 4 to 8 Fr. (1 Fr. = 0.33 mm) although larger sized sheaths are sometimes used in interventional cases. For femoral and brachial diagnostic left heart catheterizations, 6-Fr. and 5-Fr. sheaths, respectively, are most commonly used. For radial cases, a 4-Fr. or 5-Fr. dilator is frequently used prior to insertion of either a 5-Fr. or 6-Fr. sheath. In cases of severe peripheral vascular disease, a smaller dilator may need to be used initially prior to inserting a 5-Fr. or 6-Fr. system.

The length of sheaths used routinely varies from as short as 6 cm to as long as 35 cm. For most cases, an 11-cm sheath is adequate. **Longer sheaths of 25 to 35 cm are selected when one encounters tortuous femoral and/or iliac arteries in order to facilitate torque control of**

the diagnostic coronary catheter. Occasionally, with the radial approach, a longer 23-cm sheath is used to prevent radial artery spasm.

Catheter Selection: As discussed in Chapter 1, the operator should review, if available, any past coronary angiographic films to observe the catheters used for diagnostic cardiac angiography and to identify possible difficulties engaging the native coronary arteries and/or bypass grafts.

The sections of an angiographic catheter include a body (which is mostly straight throughout its course) and the tip, with various curves. The curves are classified as primary, secondary, and tertiary starting from the tip (Figure 2-1). The hub of the catheter has an airtight seal composed of a female Luer-Lok that allows attachment to a syringe or manifold, winged tips to facilitate catheter rotation, and labeling of the size of the catheter.

Diagnostic coronary catheters are sized by their external diameter, which is expressed in French sizes (1 Fr. = 0.33 mm). Most diagnostic coronary catheterizations will use 6 French (Fr.) catheters, although catheters as small as 4 Fr. and as large as 8 Fr. may occasionally be used. Catheter length varies based on the percutaneous approach and its configuration. Most pigtail catheters for ventriculography or aortography are 110 cm in length, while the commonly used Judkins catheters for coronary angiography are 100 cm long. Brachial catheters are generally 80 or 100 cm long.

Catheter selection depends upon the percutaneous approach used, whether bypass grafts are present, and coronary anatomy variations. For the left femoral, left brachial, and left radial approach, the Judkins catheters are usually the initial catheters selected. Both the left Judkins (JL) and right Judkins (JR) catheter have a primary curve of 90°. The JL has a secondary curve of 180°, while the JR has a secondary curve of 30°. The JL catheter comes in various arm (distance between the primary and secondary curve) sizes. For example, the JL4 catheter has a 4.2 cm length arm, while the JL5 and JL6 catheters have arm lengths of 5.2 and 6.2 cm, respectively. For most diagnostic cases, the JL4 catheter is attempted first. If the patient's aortic root is dilated, then a longer arm JL catheter (5 or 6) is frequently used. A smaller arm JL 3.5 catheter is chosen if the aortic root is smaller than usual, or if the left main is located superiorly. In cases where a short left main trunk is encountered, a JL4 short tip catheter usually successfully cannulates the left main ostium. If one is unable to engage the left coronary circulation with the Judkins catheters, the left Amplatz (AL) class of catheters is usually employed.

The AL catheters are particularly good at engaging a short left main trunk or in cases where the left circumflex coronary artery (LCX) and left anterior descending artery (LAD) have separate ostia. They can also

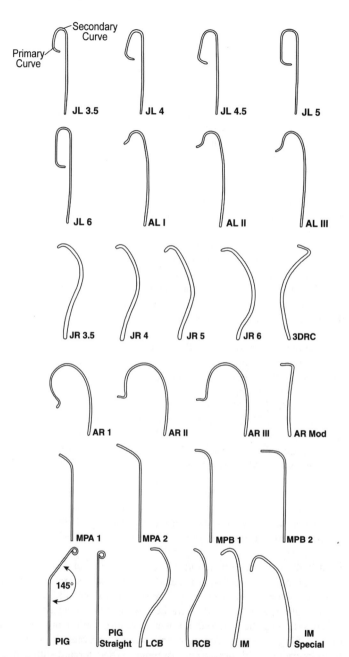

Figure **2-1** **Commonly used diagnostic catheters.** MPA, multipurpose A; MPB, multipurpose B; PIG, pigtail; LCB, left coronary bypass; RCB, right coronary bypass; IM, internal mammary; JR, Judkins right; AR, Amplatz right; AR Mod, Amplatz right modified; JL, Judkins left; AL, Amplatz left.

be used to engage high-anterior right coronary arteries (RCAs) or Shepherd's Crook RCA. The right Amplatz (AR) catheters are useful for cannulating RCAs that have an inferior orientation. Amplatz catheters are classified by the size of their secondary curve (AL1-3; AR1-3). Alternatively, a 3DRC (No Torque Right) catheter can be attempted in cases where the RCA ostium cannot be engaged with the JR4. The three-dimensional curve configuration of the 3DR catheter facilitates engagement of the RCA.

For the right arm approach (either brachial or radial), either the Amplatz, multipurpose, or modified brachial or radial catheters are commonly used. One advantage of the multipurpose catheter is that it can be used for both coronary angiography and ventriculography. The multipurpose catheter can also be used from the femoral approach, usually in cases where the RCA or left main has an inferior takeoff. Both the multipurpose and Amplatz catheters require experience for proper manipulation. **To minimize the risk of coronary dissection when using the Amplatz catheters, the operator should rotate the catheter counterclockwise to disengage it from the coronary ostium prior to removing the catheter.**

For bypass grafts, the JR4 catheter is usually successful in engaging both venous and arterial grafts. For left internal mammary artery (LIMA) or right internal mammary artery (RIMA) grafts that have a sharply angulated downward takeoff, the IMA catheter is more likely to successfully engage these grafts since it has a longer tip and less of a primary curve (80°) than the JR4. The 5-Fr. JoMed catheter is stiffer and more angulated than the IMA catheter and may be used for engaging a LIMA graft that has a sharp, downward takeoff. However, the JR4 is usually used first to engage the subclavian artery, and a long J wire is used to exchange the JR4 for the IMA catheter. For saphenous vein graft (SVG) to RCA grafts that have a steep downward orientation, the multipurpose, right bypass, or right modified Amplatz catheters can be attempted if the JR4 approach is unsuccessful. Whenever SVGs to the LAD or LCX cannot be cannulated with a JR4, one can consider alternative catheters, such as the left bypass, AL, or multipurpose.

Manifold: A variety of manifold systems exist. One common design is a three-component manifold that has three stopcocks attached. The first stopcock is connected to a pressure transducer, the second is attached to flush solution, and the third is attached to the contrast agent of choice. When setting up the manifold, it is vital to ensure that the pressure transducer tubing is flushed adequately with saline to prevent any air bubbles from interfering with pressure measurements. Shorter and stiffer tubing between the pressure transducer and catheter optimizes pressure measurements. The pressure transducer is "zeroed" with the aid of an assistant by placing the transducer at the patient's mid chest level. The stopcock to the saline port is then opened to bring down the saline through the connection tubing into the manifold. Similarly, the stopcock to the contrast agent of choice is opened and the contrast brought down to the stopcock level. The manifold is then once again flushed with saline and all tubing inspected for the presence of any air bubbles.

Vascular Access

Percutaneous Femoral Approach: The femoral approach is the most common in the United States. The operator should first identify anatomic landmarks prior to giving local anesthesia such as the inguinal ligament, which traverses from the anterior superior iliac spine to the pubic tubercle. The femoral artery generally crosses the inguinal ligament at an imaginary point that is located one third from the medial aspect and two thirds from the lateral aspect of the ligament. The femoral pulse is then palpated approximately 2 finger breadths (2–3 cm) below the inguinal ligament, marking the site of arterial access (Figure 2-2). One can also use fluoroscopy to identify femoral head. The optimal access location would be at the site over the inferior border of the femoral head. This approach is especially useful in obese patients where the identification of the inguinal ligament may be more difficult. Approximately 95% of patients have the femoral bifurcation located below the upper border of the femoral head. **Locating the optimal site of entry is important since entry sites above the inguinal ligament may lead to an increased risk of retroperitoneal bleeding, while entry sites that are too low may result in the development of arteriovenous fistula or pseudoaneurysm.**

After the entry site is determined, the femoral region is scrubbed with povidone–iodine or chlorhexidine-based solution and surgically draped. The entry site is again palpated with the index and middle fingers of the left hand either perpendicular or parallel to the artery to confirm location of the femoral pulse. With the left index and middle fingers maintaining constant moderate pressure on the artery, the operator uses his or her right hand to raise a subcutaneous wheal at the entry site with a 25-gauge needle containing roughly 3 cc of procaine 1%. A 22-gauge needle is then used to slowly deliver an additional 6 to 10 cc of local anesthetic to the deeper subcutaneous tissue. The amount of local anesthetic should cover the anticipated needle path from the skin to the artery. When giving local anesthesia, the operator should monitor the ECG monitor and the patient for any signs of a possible vagal reaction.

Holding the 18-gauge Cook access needle at the hub with the thumb and index finger, the operator inserts the needle through the skin

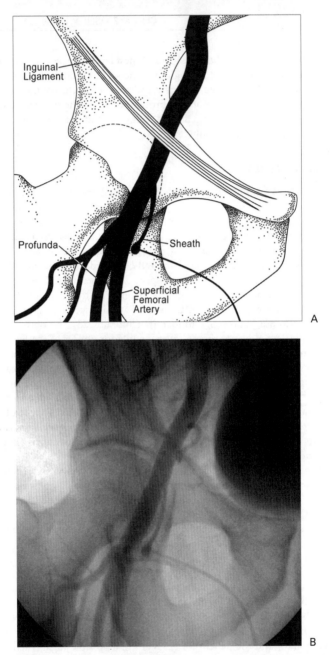

Figure **2-2** **Femoral access landmarks. A)** Diagram of femoral artery landmarks. **B)** 30° LAO projection of femoral artery. The LAO projection best displays the bifurcation of the profunda and the superficial femoral artery.

Troubleshooting

The patient is allergic to procaine: If the patient has a documented allergy to procaine (ester prototype anesthetics), then lidocaine 2% or other amide prototype local anesthetic can be given.

at a 30° to 45° angle with the bevel pointed upward. As the needle nears the femoral artery, the operator should observe the motion of the needle. A side-to-side motion usually signals that the needle is either lateral or medial to the artery, and should be repositioned. If the needle motion is up-and-down, the needle is positioned correctly, and the needle should be gently advanced. As the needle gets closer to the artery, the operator may feel arterial pulsations transmitted through the needle hub. Brisk, pulsatile blood return signals successful arterial puncture. A 45-cm J-tipped 0.035-cm guidewire is then advanced through the needle. The needle is removed, and a small nick is made at the level of the skin with a scalpel to facilitate insertion of the sheath size of choice (usually 6 Fr.) over the guidewire. The dilator within the sheath and the guidewire are subsequently removed and the sheath flushed with saline. The arterial pressure should then be documented by attaching the side port of the sheath to the manifold.

Arm Approaches: In cases of morbid obesity, severe peripheral vascular disease, aortic dissection, or aortic aneurysm, the femoral approach is either very difficult or contraindicated. If coronary angiography is indicated, the brachial or radial approaches are used. Because the brachial and radial arteries are smaller caliber vessels, heparin (3,000–5,000 units IV) should be used to avoid arterial thrombosis. Right brachial or radial arterial access has the advantage of allowing the operator to remain on the right side of the catheterization table to manipulate and exchange catheters and to access the table and fluoroscopy controls. It has the disadvantage of often requiring specialized catheters for cannulation of the coronary ostia, and precludes injection of the left subclavian artery or LIMA, which is necessary if the LIMA is used as a coronary bypass graft. Access via the left brachial or radial artery allows the operator to use standard femoral catheters (such as the Judkins catheters) for cannulation of the coronary ostia and allows selective engagement of the LIMA. Manipulation and exchange of catheters is more difficult, however, because of the distance of the access point from the operator.

Percutaneous Brachial Approach: Prior to local anesthesia, the brachial and radial pulses of both arms should be palpated. The Allen test should

Poor blood return: Weak blood flow may signal that the needle may be located against the vessel wall, subintimally, or in a smaller branch. Gentle forward or backward manipulation or a slight change in the angulation of the needle may improve blood flow. Alternatively, sluggish blood flow may be secondary to severe peripheral vascular disease or low perfusion states.

There is resistance advancing the guidewire: The guidewire should only be inserted through the needle when brisk, pulsatile blood flow is obtained. If resistance is encountered as the guidewire is passing through the tip of the needle that is not relieved by reducing the angle of the needle, the guidewire should be removed and brisk pulsatile blood flow should be confirmed. If blood flow is not brisk, the needle may be gently redirected in an attempt to restore blood flow. If these maneuvers are unsuccessful, the needle should be removed and pressure held over the entry site for 5 minutes before reattempting access. If resistance is encountered or the patient begins to complain of pain after the guidewire has been successfully advanced a few centimeters, then fluoroscopy should be used to document location of the guidewire. In this situation, the needle is removed, and a small sheath (5 Fr.) can be carefully advanced to the point where resistance was encountered. The wire is then removed and the sheath aspirated to confirm blood return and flushed. Using a small amount (5 cc) of either nonionic or diluted ionic contrast, the operator then injects contrast under fluoroscopy to assess for arterial dissection, vessel tortuosity, or severe atherosclerosis.

A retrograde subintimal dissection is found after access is secured: Subintimal retrograde dissections caused by guidewire insertions rarely cause arterial complications. The patient should be monitored closely for signs and symptoms of dissection extension (progressive pain, pale extremities, loss of distal pulses). Either the other femoral artery, or a brachial or radial approach should be accessed for left heart catheterization.

Severe vessel tortuosity or atherosclerosis is encountered: Reinserting a softer, more steerable guidewire (Wholey) or hydrophilic-coated guidewire (Glidewire) may enable passage through the tortuosity or stenosis. A long sheath (45-cm Arrow or 55-cm Brite Tip long sheath) should be considered to improve catheter manipulation.

Resistance during sheath placement is encountered: Confirm that an adequate nick has been made at the level of the skin. Resistance may also originate from severe vessel calcification or scar tissue from prior procedures. Using first a smaller dilator (4 or 5 Fr.) to predilate along with a stiffer wire (0.038 cm or Amplatz wire) may facilitate placement of the sheath.

Femoral pulse is not easily palpable: One could attempt using the Smart Needle device. With this device, the needle is directed to the site where the arterial pulsations are heard best via the Doppler probe.

Patient has prosthetic femoral artery grafts: If the vascular graft is older than 2 to 3 months, then the percutaneous femoral approach can be considered. Predilation with a smaller dilator is recommended prior to insertion of the desired sheath size to prevent the sheath from kinking as it passes through the graft.

also be performed. The brachial artery is approximately 3 to 5 mm in diameter. The strongest brachial pulse is generally located 1 to 2 cm above the elbow crease. The antecubital fossa is then sterilized and draped. Using a 25-gauge needle, a small wheal is raised using approximately 3 cc of local anesthetic. Injecting larger amounts of local anesthetic may make it more difficult to palpate the brachial pulse. One can use either an 18-gauge needle or a micropuncture needle (22-gauge) to obtain arterial access using a 45° angle. With the micropuncture needle kit, a stiffer 0.025 guidewire is used, while the standard 0.035-cm guidewire is used for the 18-gauge needle. Once the guidewire is inserted into the artery, a 5-Fr. or 6-Fr. sheath is usually inserted as described in the percutaneous femoral approach. Heparin 3,000 to 5,000 units IV should be considered to avoid sheath thrombosis.

Percutaneous Radial Approach: As described with the brachial approach, the Allen test should be performed prior to radial artery catheterization. The patient's arm is abducted at a 70° angle and the wrist is hyperextended. Topical anesthetic cream is then applied over the radial artery to reduce the amount of local anesthetic needed after the area is cleaned in a sterile fashion and draped. Local anesthesia is then given as depicted in the brachial approach. Next, either an 18-gauge needle or a micropuncture needle (22-gauge) is inserted at a 30° to 45° angle approximately 1 cm from the styloid process. The guidewire is then advanced as described in the brachial approach. A 4-Fr. or 5-Fr. dilator is then used to predilate the radial artery. A 5-Fr. or 6-Fr. sheath is then inserted over a standard 0.035-cm guidewire. A longer sheath (23 cm) may be used in radial cases to decrease radial artery spasm. Alternatively, standard sheath lengths may be used with local infusions of nitroglycerine or verapamil. Heparin 3,000 to 5,000 units IV should be considered to avoid sheath thrombosis.

Suggested Reading

Bashore TM, Bates ER, Berger PB, et al. American College of Cardiology/Society for Cardiac Angiography and Interventions Clinical Expert Consensus Document on cardiac catheterization laboratory standards. A report of the American College of Cardiology Task Force on Clinical Expert Consensus Documents. *J Am Coll Cardiol.* 2001;37(8):2170–2214.

Davidson C, Stacul F, McCullough PA, et al. Contrast medium use. *Am J Cardiol.* 2006;98(6A):42K–58K.

Denys BG, Uretsky BF, Baughman K, et al. Accessing vascular structures. In: Uretsky BF, ed. *Cardiac Catheterization: Concepts, Techniques and Applications.* Malden: Blackwell Science; 1997:93–118.

Einstein AJ, Moser KW, Thompson RC, et al. Radiation dose to patients from cardiac diagnostic imaging. *Circulation.* 2007;116(11):1290–1305.

Limacher MC, Douglas PS, Germano G, et al. ACC expert consensus document. Radiation safety in the practice of cardiology. American College of Cardiology. *J Am Coll Cardiol.* 1998;31(4):892–913.

McCullough PA. Contrast-induced acute kidney injury. *J Am Coll Cardiol.* 2008;51(15):1419–1428.

Meth MJ, Maibach HI. Current understanding of contrast media reactions and implications for clinical management. *Drug Saf.* 2006;29(2):133–141.

Wagner LK, Archer BR. *Minimizing Risks from Fluoroscopic X-Rays: Bioeffects, Instrumentation, and Examination.* 3rd ed. Houston: Partners in Radiation Management; 2000.

Universal Protocol for Disease Specific Care. The Joint Commission. Available at: http://www.jointcommission.org/PatientSafety/UniversalProtocol/. Accessed May 2, 2009.

CHAPTER 3

Native Coronary Angiography

Stephen Gimple, Niranjan Seshadri,
Robert E. Hobbs, and Sorin Brener

The coronary arteries arise from the sinuses of Valsalva. The left main coronary artery arises from the left sinus. After a short course, the left main trunk usually bifurcates into the left anterior descending and left circumflex coronary arteries. In some instances, it may trifurcate, with the ramus intermedius being the intermediate vessel in the trifurcation. The current classification of coronary anatomy is based on the CASS system.

The left anterior descending artery (LAD) follows a course along the anterior interventricular groove to the apex of the heart, supplying blood to the anterior wall, the septum via septal perforators and the anterolateral wall via diagonal branches.

The left circumflex coronary artery (LCX) courses along the left atrioventricular groove supplying the lateral wall of the left ventricle. The branches arising from the left circumflex are called obtuse marginals, with the first branch arising from the atrioventricular circumflex called obtuse marginal 1, the second branch called obtuse marginal 2, and so forth.

The right coronary artery (RCA) arises from the right sinus of Valsalva and travels along the right atrioventricular groove. The first branch that arises from the right coronary artery is the conus branch, which supplies the right ventricular outflow tract. In approximately 50% of the cases, the conus branch has a separate origin. Localizing the conus branch may be important in selected cases because it is often a critical source of collateral circulation to the LAD. Other branches include the artery to the sinus node, which arises from the RCA in 60% of cases; the acute marginal branches, which supply the right ventricle; the artery to the AV node; the diaphragmatic artery; and terminal branches: the posteroventricular branches and the posterior descending artery (PDA) in most cases.

The PDA, which courses in the posterior interventricular groove, determines coronary dominance. In 85% of the cases, the PDA arises from the RCA, making the coronary circulation right dominant. In 7% of the cases, the circulation is codominant, with the posterior interventricular groove being supplied by both the RCA and the LCX. In 8% of the cases, the PDA arises from the left circumflex making it the dominant artery.

Engaging the Coronary Arteries

For diagnostic coronary angiography, we routinely use 4 or 5 Fr. Judkins left and right catheters via the femoral approach. However, the use of the radial approach in appropriately selected patients is increasing and may soon be the standard for diagnostic angiography. Use of smaller caliber 4 or 5 Fr. systems has some advantages. For example, in patients requiring only diagnostic angiography prior to heart valve surgery, use of a 4-Fr. system decreases recovery time and allows faster ambulation after sheath removal (see Chapter 8). In addition, the use of the radial approach also fosters shorter recovery times as well as shorter hospitalization times.

Engaging the Left Coronary System: Assuming that the size of the aorta is within normal limits, a Judkins left 4 (JL4) is routinely used. The catheters are flushed with heparinized saline and advanced over a J-tipped guide wire ("J wire") through the femoral sheath and to the ascending aorta just above the aortic root. **To avoid retrograde dissection of the aorta, catheters are advanced with the J-tipped guide wire protruding beyond the proximal end of the catheter**. Once the catheter is just above the sinus of Valsalva, the guide wire is withdrawn and a few drops of blood are allowed to back bleed from the catheter allowing for clearance of debris that may have collected during catheter advancement. The catheter is then connected to the manifold, flushed with saline, and the syringe is loaded with dye. Once an adequate pressure tracing is seen, the catheter is opacified with 1 to 2 cc of contrast dye and is ready for selective engagement.

Using the Judkins technique, not much effort is required to cannulate the ostium of the left main trunk. The catheter is advanced into the aortic root, and in the majority of the patients, it will engage the ostium. The catheter tip should be coaxial with the left main trunk. In cases where the left main trunk is not easily cannulated, a clockwise or a counterclockwise turn may help engage the ostium.

Once the ostium of the left main trunk is engaged, a good pressure waveform should be observed before proceeding with coronary arteriography.

The catheter does not back bleed: If the catheter does not back bleed after removing the guidewire, the tip may be apposed to the wall of the aorta. Gently withdraw the catheter, and turn it either clockwise or counterclockwise to free the catheter tip. After discarding a few drops of blood, connect the catheter hub to the manifold and look at the pressure tracing.

No waveform is observed in the pressure tracing: If no waveform is observed in the pressure tracing, the transducer may not be opened to pressure. This may be rectified by manipulating the first of the three-way stopcocks on the manifold or by turning the transducer at the side of the table to the on position.

Catheter is NOT engaged and the waveform is dampened: This may be due to air in the system or the catheter may be partially against the arterial wall. To eliminate air in the system, first gently withdraw a few drops of blood and flush the manifold and catheter with saline, taking care not to reintroduce air in the system. A gentle clockwise or counterclockwise rotation along with pulling back the catheter will move the tip away from the aortic wall. If the dampened waveform persists, it may be due to air in the pressure transducer tubing. Flush the transducer tubing and recheck the pressure. If the problem persists, in rare cases, the catheter itself may have a kink, in which case it needs to be replaced.

The aorta is dilated, and it is difficult to engage the left main trunk with the JL4: In the case of a dilated aorta, the curve on the JL4 catheter may be too short to engage the ostium of the left main trunk. Upsizing to a JL5 or even JL6 catheter may help. Additionally, with a dilated aorta there may not be a hinge point for the arm of the catheter to rest. In this case, a counterclockwise (moves the catheter anteriorly) or a clockwise rotation (moves the catheter posteriorly) helps engage the ostium.

The patient is not of average height: The size of the aorta is often proportional to the height of the patient. Some operators start with a JL4 in nearly all patients. Other operators will start with a JL3.5 if the patient is less than 5′4″ tall, or a JL5 if the patient is greater than 6′2″ tall.

The left main trunk has an unusual takeoff: In some cases, the ostium of the left main trunk may have a takeoff in a plane that may be out of the reach of the Judkins catheters (usually a high posterior origin). Switching to an Amplatz system may be helpful. Amplatz catheters are advanced around the aortic arch over a guide wire. The catheter is further advanced until the curve rests in the left sinus of Valsalva with the tip facing the ostium of the left main trunk. Withdrawal and gentle clockwise and/or counterclockwise rotation brings the tip in plane with the coronary ostia. To disengage the Amplatz catheter, it is important to first push it gently forward (brings the tip out of the coronary ostium), and rotate before pulling back, all under fluoroscopic guidance.

Troubleshooting

The catheter is engaged and the waveform is dampened: A dampened pressure waveform (drop in the catheter tip systolic pressure) or a ventricularized pressure waveform (drop in the catheter tip diastolic pressure) usually indicates that the catheter tip is either deep seated, restricting coronary inflow, or the tip is against the wall. It also indicates the possibility of significant left main stenosis. This can be a dangerous situation that needs to be recognized quickly. The catheter tip should be immediately withdrawn from the ostium. The ostium can be re-engaged cautiously. If a small injection of dye reveals significant ostial left main stenosis (another clue may be the absence of dye reflux into the aortic root with the injection), two short cine runs aimed at visualizing distal targets for bypass surgery should promptly be performed, and the catheter then immediately pulled back from the ostium. Care must be taken to avoid multiple engagements of the left main trunk as this can lead to abrupt vessel closure. In cases where significant left main trunk stenosis is suspected, the operator can take nonselective angiograms of the left main trunk by injecting dye with the catheter tip positioned in left sinus. Catheter damping may also be seen in cases of spasm of the left main trunk. In such instances, intracoronary nitroglycerin can be injected (200 μg) and follow-up picture can be taken to document relief of spasm.

Engaging the Right Coronary Artery: Engaging the RCA often requires more skill with catheter manipulation than engaging the left coronary artery. The Judkins right 4 (JR4) catheter is most commonly used. The JR4 is advanced to the right coronary cusp, with the tip facing the left ostium. The catheter is gently pulled back while simultaneously rotating the catheter clockwise to engage the right ostium (the tip of the catheter tends to migrate down toward the sinuses with clockwise rotation). Alternatively, the clockwise rotation may be performed above the plane of the right coronary ostium without pulling back. This will make the catheter tip move down toward the sinus while rotating. The ostium is usually found about 2 cm above the aortic valve. After engaging, the pressure waveform is visualized, and if satisfactory, coronary arteriography may be performed.

Coronary Angiographic Views

Coronary arteriography provides a silhouette of the epicardial coronary arteries. The basic views, posteroanterior (PA), left anterior oblique (LAO), right anterior oblique (RAO) with or without varying degrees of either cranial or caudal angulation, show the coronaries in orthogonal views, while minimizing interference by other structures, such as the

Troubleshooting

Difficulty engaging the RCA: The ostium may be high and anterior, posterior, or angled upwardly. A 3DR catheter may be used if the JR4 catheter fails to engage the ostium. This catheter is dropped to the aortic valve and gently pulled back without rotating the catheter. For a high and anterior takeoff (frequently seen in transplanted hearts due to rotation of the heart), pulling the catheter further back with a less clockwise turn usually engages the ostium. For a posteriorly directed ostium, further clockwise rotation may be required. For an upwardly directed ostium or dilated ascending aorta, an Amplatz catheter works well. To engage the ostium of the RCA arising from the left sinus of Valsalva, an Amplatz left (AL 1) catheter may be used. Other catheters that may be used include an Amplatz right or a multipurpose catheter.

The pressure waveform is dampened or ventricularized: This usually indicates the catheter tip is either deep seated, restricting coronary inflow; the tip is against the wall; the conus branch is selectively engaged; or there may be spasm or severe disease of the ostium. If the catheter tip is too far in the artery, the catheter is withdrawn gently without disengaging the ostium and a gentle counter clockwise rotation usually stabilizes the catheter. A gentle clockwise or counterclockwise rotation moves the tip away from the ostium. If the conus branch has a separate ostium, then the catheter may need to be slightly repositioned to avoid this branch, as the main RCA ostium is often very close in proximity. If spasm is suspected, a gentle test injection is performed. The catheter is disengaged, gently re-engaged, and intracoronary nitroglycerin or a sublingual nitroglycerin is administered, provided the blood pressure is acceptable and the image remains suspicious for spasm. If there is true ostial narrowing, a quick injection with just enough dye to fill the artery is done and the catheter is removed from the ostium. Failure to promptly remove the catheter from the ostium of the artery, or proceeding with angiography in the presence of a dampened waveform increases the risk of inducing ventricular fibrillation. Ostial spasm usually occurs a few seconds after engaging the artery. This helps differentiate it from a fixed stenosis.

Torque buildup: When a catheter is rotated from outside the sheath, the torque must be transmitted to the catheter tip before it will rotate. This is best accomplished by gently and quickly moving the catheter in and out a few millimeters while rotating. If torque is allowed to build up within the catheter, the tip can suddenly spin, or "helicopter," which could cause disruption of aortic plaque or potentially even coronary dissection. Torque buildup is often more problematic in patients with very tortuous iliacs and aortas. Placing a longer sheath can often improve rotational control of the catheter.

spine and the diaphragm. It is important that each segment of coronary is evaluated in two orthogonal views, with care to avoid significant vessel overlap and with visualization of all important side branches.

In the LAO projection, the image intensifier (II) is to the left of the patient. On fluoroscopy, the spine is to the right of the screen in an LAO view. In the RAO projection, the II is to the right of the patient and the spine is on the left of the screen in fluoroscopy. In general, cranial angulation is ideal for visualizing the distal portion of vessels, and caudal angulation is ideal for visualizing the proximal portion of vessels. The commonly used views shown in Table 3-1 represent only a guide and need to be modified for each individual patient.

During cine runs, patients should be instructed to take in and hold a deep breath, especially with cranial angulations, to move the diaphragm out of view as far as possible.

Left Coronary System Views: The first view of the left coronary system should delineate the course of the left main coronary trunk. Most operators prefer either a straight PA or a 20° RAO and 20° caudal angulation (Figure 3-1). The spine should be off the origin of the left main coronary trunk.

The 20° RAO, 20° caudal view is an ideal view for the proximal circumflex. In this view, while panning down the circumflex, portions of the LAD may also be visualized. The operator can also visualize the LCX artery using a straight PA 30° caudal view.

A straight PA 40° cranial angulation view highlights the mid and distal portions of the LAD (Figure 3-2). To separate out the diagonals from

Table **3-1**	Commonly Used Angiographic Views
	Vessel Optimally Viewed
Left Coronary Artery	
20° RAO, 20° caudal	LMT and LCX
40° PA cranial	LAD
45° LAO, 30° cranial	LAD and diagonals
30° RAO, 30° cranial	LAD
45° LAO, 30° caudal	LMT, proximal LAD, and proximal LCX
Right Coronary Artery	
40° LAO	Proximal and mid RCA
40° PA cranial	Distal RCA (PDA and PV branches)
35° RAO	Proximal and mid RCA

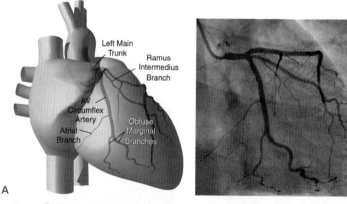

Figure **3-1   20° RAO–20° caudal view of the left coronary artery. A)** 3D diagram of the 20° RAO–20° caudal view. **B)** Angiogram of the 20° RAO–20° caudal view. This view is optimal for visualization of the left main trunk and the left circumflex arteries. Note that the left circumflex artery courses posterior to the heart in this view, a detail best appreciated in the 3D diagram. As in all RAO views, the spine and the diagnostic catheter lie to the left of the heart.

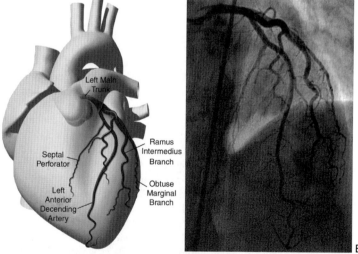

Figure **3-2   40° PA cranial view of the left coronary artery. A)** 3D diagram of the 40° PA cranial view. **B)** Angiogram of the 40° PA cranial view. This view is optimal for visualization of the mid and distal portion of the left anterior descending artery and proximal portion of all diagonal branches.

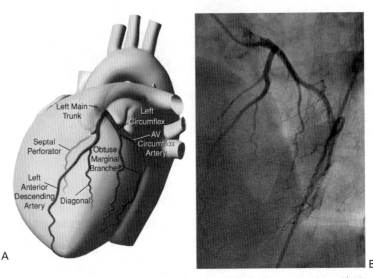

A

B

Figure **3-3**   **45° LAO–20° cranial view of the left coronary artery. A)** 3D diagram of the 45° LAO–20° cranial view. **B)** Angiogram of the 45° LAO–20° cranial view. This view is optimal for visualization of the left anterior descending and the entire length of the diagonal branches. As in all LAO views, the catheter and the spine are to the right of the heart.

the LAD, a 30° RAO with a 25° to 30° cranial angulation is used. The diagonals are placed above the LAD in this view. Other useful views to separate the diagonals from the LAD are the 40° to 50° LAO and the 25° to 30° cranial views (Figure 3-3).

The proximal LAD and the left main coronary artery can also be visualized using the 45° LAO and 30° caudal view (Figure 3-4). This view is also known as the "spider view." The origins of the LCX and the proximal diagonals are also well seen.

In cases where the mid-LAD needs to be visualized in additional views, such as would be the case for LIMA graft insertions, the straight lateral view 90° LAO is very useful.

Right Coronary Artery Views: The RCA is viewed in either a straight RAO or LAO (35–40°) view (Figure 3-5) or a PA view with cranial angulation. The 40° LAO view shows the ostium, proximal, and mid portions best (Figure 3-6), but the PDA and the posteroventricular branches are also well visualized.

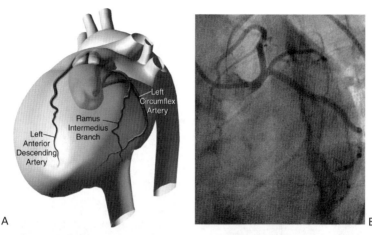

Figure **3-4**   **50° LAO–35° caudal view of the left coronary artery ("spider view"). A)** 3D diagram of the 50° LAO–35° caudal view. **B)** Angiogram of the 50° LAO–35° caudal view. This view is optimal for visualization of the left main trunk and the proximal portions of the left anterior descending and the left circumflex arteries. In cases of occlusion of the right coronary artery, it is important to maintain cine long enough to visualize the extent of potential collaterals to the right coronary artery.

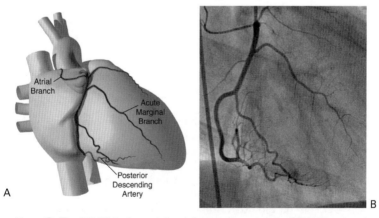

Figure **3-5**   **30° RAO view of the right coronary artery. A)** 3D diagram of the 35° RAO view. **B)** Angiogram of the 35° RAO view. This view is best for visualization of the posterior descending branch of the right coronary artery.

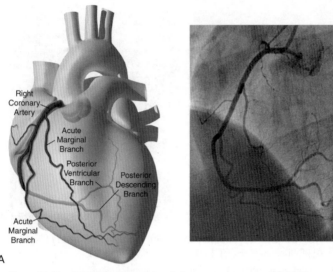

Figure **3-6** **35° LAO view of the right coronary artery. A)** 3D diagram of the 35° LAO view. **B)** Angiogram of the 35° LAO view. The posterior descending artery branch in this view is typically the most inferior vessel arising from the distal right coronary artery. In cases of severe obstructions of the left anterior descending artery, it is important to maintain cine long enough to visualize collaterals from the distal right coronary artery or from the conus branch to the left anterior descending artery.

The bifurcation of the RCA, PDA, and the posteroventricular branches are best seen in the 40° PA cranial view.

Coronary Anomalies

The various coronary anomalies in order of frequency are listed below:

- Left anterior descending and left circumflex arteries arising from separate ostia (0.5%) (Figure 3-7)
- Origin of the LCX from the right sinus of Valsalva (0.5%) (Figure 3-8)
- Origin of the RCA from the ascending aorta above the right sinus of Valsalva (0.2%) (Figure 3-9)
- Origin of the RCA from the left sinus of Valsalva (0.1%) (Figure 3-10)
- AV fistula (0.1%) (Figure 3-11)
- Origin of the left main trunk from the right sinus of Valsalva (0.02%) (Figure 3-12)

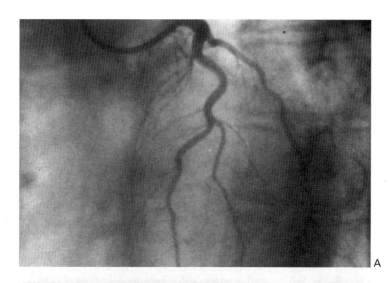

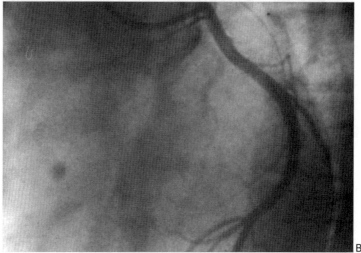

Figure **3-7**   **Left anterior descending and left circumflex arteries arise from separate orifices.** Panels **A** and **B** show selective engagement of the left anterior descending and the left circumflex artery. *(continued)*

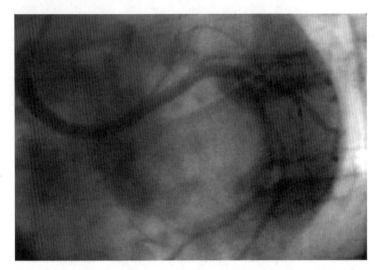

Figure **3-8** **Left circumflex artery arising from the right sinus of Valsalva.**
LAO projection of anomalous circumflex from right sinus of Valsalva passes inferior and posterior to aorta where it reaches the left atrioventricular groove and distributes normally over the lateral wall of the heart. In the LAO projection, this anomaly has the appearance of the letter "S" or "question mark" on its side.

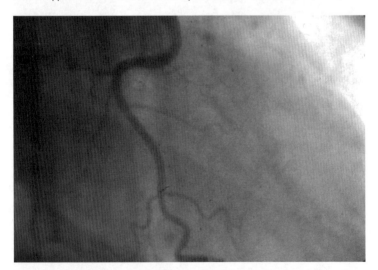

Figure **3-9** **Right coronary artery arising from the ascending aorta above the right sinus of Valsalva.** Right coronary artery arises from the ascending aorta above the right sinus of Valsalva, RAO projection. Note that the initial segment of this vessel is vertically oriented.

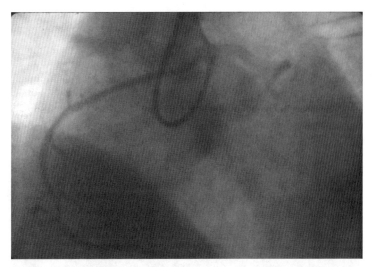

Figure **3-10** **Right coronary artery arising from the left sinus of Valsalva.** Anomalous right coronary artery arises from the left sinus of Valsalva passing between the aorta and the pulmonary artery and to the right atrioventricular groove before distributing normally, LAO projection. Patients with this anomaly are at increased risk for sudden death, and it requires surgical correction.

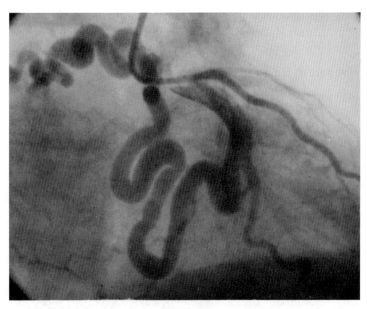

Figure **3-11** **AV fistula arising from left circumflex artery draining into superior vena cava.** Serpiginous course of an AV fistula arising from left circumflex artery and draining into the superior vena cava, RAO projection.

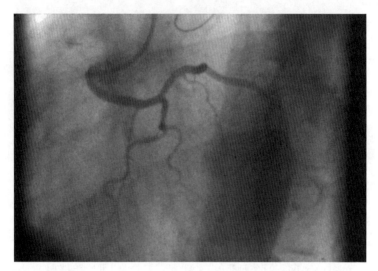

Figure **3-12**   **Left main trunk arising from the right sinus of Valsalva.**
Anomalous origin of the LMT from the right sinus of Valsalva. Selective visualization of the left coronary artery, LAO projection. The LMT arises from the right
sinus of Valsalva and passes into the interventricular septum where it gives off a
septal perforator. The vessel then reaches the epicardial surface of the heart
where it divides into the LAD and LCX which distribute normally.

Myocardial Bridging

In myocardial bridging, portions of epicardial coronary arteries (most
commonly the LAD and the diagonals) run within the myocardium
(Figure 3-13). Obliteration of the coronary lumen during systole with resolution in diastole may be seen. Because the majority of myocardial blood
flow occurs in diastole, most cases of bridging are clinically benign (98%
11-year survival). However, in rare situations, myocardial bridges may be
associated with angina, myocardial ischemia, myocardial infarction, left
ventricular dysfunction, myocardial stunning, paroxysmal AV blockade,
exercise-induced ventricular tachycardia, or sudden cardiac death.
Effective therapies include beta-blockade, and in severe cases, coronary
stenting or surgical myotomy with or without concomitant bypass surgery.

Image Quality

Due to the invasive nature of the study, and to the important decisions
made with the information, it is vital to obtain high-quality images
when performing coronary angiography. A host of factors are involved

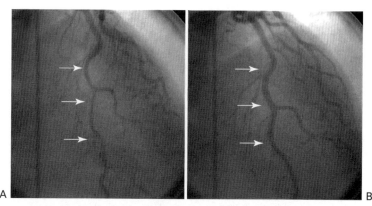

A B

Figure **3-13** **Myocardial bridging.** Hypertrophied myocardium compressing the mid portion of the left anterior descending artery during **A)** systole *(arrows)*. Resolution of arterial compression during **B)** diastole *(arrows)*.

with the quality of the image, including patient issues and operator technique.

Patient Factors: Patients who are obese provide lower-quality images due to difficulty with x-ray penetration. The dose of radiation may be increased in these patients to improve image quality at the expense of greater radiation exposure. Bone is dense, and images are of better quality when the coronaries are not superimposed over the spine. Changing the amount of lateral angulation can move the spine away from the area of interest. The density of the diaphragm also creates shadowing which degrades image quality. Patients should be asked to take and hold a deep breath, especially during cranial views, to drop the diaphragm out of view. The lungs are very radiolucent, and look very bright on cine, causing "washout." Shielding should be used to cover the lung fields.

Operator Technique: Before a good cineangiogram can be taken, the vessel must be adequately engaged in a coaxial orientation. A catheter that does not properly fit in the vessel is either a danger for dissection or will not allow for adequate filling of the vessel with contrast. The force with which the contrast is injected is also important. Flow must be ramped up to avoid blowing the catheter out of the vessel, and injection must be sufficiently strong to prevent streaming within the artery which will make the angiogram nondiagnostic. The goal of panning during cineangiography is to visualize the arteries with as little movement as possible. Cine should begin two cardiac cycles prior to injection to look for calcification and to see other hardware or foreign bodies, and cine should continue long enough to evaluate for any late collateral vessels.

Complications of Native Coronary Angiography

Coronary angiography is a safe procedure. The overall risk of major complications (death, myocardial infarction, significant embolization) is less than 0.1%. It is important to understand potential complications so that they can be avoided when possible.

Vascular complications are the most common complications of cardiac catheterizations. These include hematoma, pseudoaneurysm, arteriovenous fistula formation, retroperitoneal bleeding, and vascular occlusion. Precise placement of the sheath below the inguinal ligament and above the bifurcation of the femoral artery will decrease retroperitoneal bleeds, pseudoanuerysms, and AV fistulas. Meticulous care in insertion and removal of the arterial sheath is necessary to minimize bleeding and vessel injury (see Chapters 2 and 9 for more information).

Aortic Dissection: Iatrogenic retrograde dissection is largely preventable with careful catheter manipulation. The J-tipped guide wire should always protrude beyond the tip of the catheter during advancement. Catheters and wires should never be advanced against resistance. The tip of the guide wire should be seen by fluoroscopy during advancement to avoid branch vessel engagement (with special care to avoid the carotid arteries). Fortunately, most retrograde dissections are non–flow limiting and self-limited and will seal on their own. However, vascular repair is occasionally needed.

Coronary Dissection: Injection of contrast when the catheter is against the wall of the coronary artery (ventricularization of the pressure waveform may give a clue to this) may result in coronary dissection. With a dissection, contrast is not cleared from the artery wall after termination of the injection (Figure 3-14). Coronary dissection can also occur from forceful engagement of the catheter into the coronary ostium. Prompt percutaneous repair or coronary bypass surgery should be considered.

Coronary spasm can occur anywhere within the coronary tree. During angiography, spasm may be induced at the coronary ostium due to mechanical irritation from the catheter tip. The catheter should be disengaged and very gently re-engaged. Intracoronary nitroglycerin should be injected into the vessel. It is most important to differentiate spasm from ostial atherosclerotic plaque. Spasm should be suspected if the vessel initially appears normal in caliber, but on subsequent views appears to

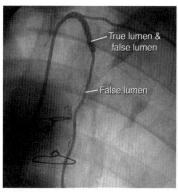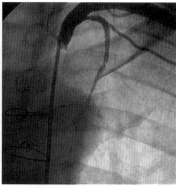

Figure **3-14   Iatrogenic dissection of a left internal mammary graft.**
A) Dissection of left internal mammary graft showing both the true and false lumen. The thicker proximal segment represents the true lumen plus the false lumen (*large arrows*), and the thinner distal segment represents the false dissecting lumen (*small arrows*). **B)** Next run shows thrombosed graft with absence of blood flow.

be stenotic, or if a severe, smooth, ostial stenosis is seen in an otherwise normal-appearing coronary.

Air Embolism: While performing coronary arteriography, extreme caution should be exercised to avoid inadvertently injecting air into the coronary arteries. To prevent this, all air should be removed from the manifold and tubing system after each hookup of the catheter. The manifold should be held at a 45° angle or greater during injection so that any unrecognized bubbles remain in the syringe. If air is injected into a coronary artery, the patient may develop chest pain with or without ST segment elevation on the ECG monitor, or ventricular fibrillation as a complication. Saline and intracoronary nitroglycerin should be repeatedly injected into the coronary artery to clear the air emboli.

Suggested Reading

Bashore TM, Bates ER, Berger PB, et al. American College of Cardiology/ Society for Cardiac Angiography and Interventions clinical expert consensus document on cardiac catheterization laboratory standards. *J Am Coll Cardiol.* 2001;37:2170–2214.

Baum S. *Abram's Angiography.* 4th ed. Boston: Little, Brown and Company; 1997:241–252.

Ellis SG. Coronary angiography. In: Fuster V, Ross R, Topol E, eds. *Atherosclerosis and Coronary Artery Disease*. Vol 2. Philadelphia: Lippincott–Raven Publishers; 1996:1433–1450.

Green CE. *Coronary Cinematography*. Philadelphia: Lippincott–Raven Publishers; 1996:39–68.

Heupler FA, Proudfit WL, Razavi M, et al. Ergonovine maleate provocative test for coronary arterial spasm. *Am J Cardiol*. 1978;41:631–640.

Manske CL, Sprafka JM, Strony JT, et al. Contrast nephropathy in azotemic diabetic patients undergoing coronary angiography. *Am J Med*. 1990;89: 615–620.

Matthai WH, Kussmal WG, Krol J, et al. A comparison of low- with high-osmolar contrast agents in cardiac angiography: identification of criteria for selective use. *Circulation*. 1994;89:291–301.

Tilkian AG, Daily EK. *Cardiovascular Procedures: Diagnostic Techniques and Therapeutic Procedures*. St. Louis: Mosby; 1986:117–151.

Yamanaka O, Hobbs RE. Coronary artery anomalies in 126,595 patients undergoing coronary arteriography. *Catheter Cardiovasc Diagn*. 1990;21:28–40.

CHAPTER 4

Bypass Graft Angiography

Kellan E. Ashley

Selective angiography of saphenous vein and arterial bypass grafts is usually performed immediately after angiography of the native coronary arteries. The technique for bypass graft opacification is similar to that employed for native coronary artery angiography. Knowledge of common graft locations and familiarity with multiple catheter types are essential to perform a complete study.

Saphenous Vein Grafts

Saphenous veins are the most commonly employed conduits in coronary revascularization. Approximately 87% of saphenous vein grafts (SVGs) remain patent at 6 months, with the patency rates dropping to approximately 63% at 10 years. Because of the high incidence of graft attrition, repeat revascularization often becomes necessary, requiring coronary angiography to assess graft patency.

The proximal anastomosis of most aortocoronary SVGs lies on the anterior surface of the aorta, several centimeters above the sinuses of Valsalva. Usually, the location of the various grafts in relation to one another follows a predictable sequence. Grafts to the left circumflex coronary artery (LCX) are typically placed most superior, followed in succession inferiorly by grafts to the diagonal branches of the left anterior descending artery (LAD), the LAD itself, and the right coronary artery (RCA) (Figure 4-1). It should be noted, however, that because of variations in surgical technique, exceptions to this rule commonly exist. **If prior angiograms are available, they should be reviewed firsthand prior to diagnostic angiography, as these can be extremely helpful in locating graft ostia and for selection of catheters.**

The Judkins right 4 (JR4) catheter is the most common catheter employed in pursuit of vein grafts. **Typically, grafts to the RCA can be best visualized and cannulated while in the left anterior oblique (LAO) projection, while grafts to the left coronary artery (LCA)**

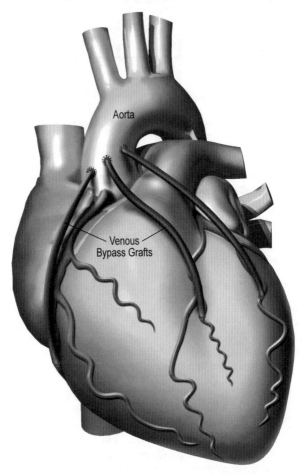

Figure **4-1** **Three-dimensional diagram illustrating the usual surgical placement of saphenous vein grafts.** From superior to inferior in the aorta, the grafts anastomose to the lateral circumflex (obtuse marginal), diagonal, and right coronary arteries.

system are most easily found while in the right anterior oblique (RAO) projection (Table 4-1). The proximal anastomosis sites of these grafts lie superior to the native coronary ostia. Some surgeons place ostial graft markers on the outer surface of the aorta at the time of surgery to facilitate location of the grafts during future catheterizations. Surgical clips may also provide clues as to the location of grafts.

Table **4-1**	General Graft Views		
Graft	**Ostium and Body**	**Distal Anastomosis**	**Native Artery**
LIMA → LAD or SVG → LAD	Straight LAO and RAO	Left lateral view; LAO cranial	PA cranial
SVG → Diagonal	Straight LAO and RAO	RAO cranial	LAO cranial
SVG → LCX	Straight LAO and RAO	RAO caudal	RAO caudal
SVG → RCA	Straight LAO and RAO	LAO	PA cranial

Steady "up and down" movements of the catheter in the ascending aorta with slight clockwise or counterclockwise rotations, typically from the second to the fourth sternal sutures, facilitate engagement of the various grafts. The catheter tip often "jumps" forward when it cannulates a graft ostium. Damping of the pressure waveform may indicate that the catheter tip is lying against the vessel wall or that there is an ostial stenosis. In this situation, the catheter should be cautiously withdrawn while simultaneously reversing its torque. Occasionally, the pressure waveform remains damped, and it may be necessary to perform a ramped injection of contrast with quick removal of the catheter in order to rule out critical stenosis or subtotal obstruction of a graft. Remember that injecting through a deep-seated catheter may not define an ostial stenosis. Occluded grafts will appear as a "stump" upon selective injection.

If a graft cannot be cannulated, do not assume that the graft is occluded. Other catheters with different angulation may be necessary. **If further attempts fail, aortography via a pigtail catheter may be helpful in locating difficult-to-find grafts.** To locate bypass grafts to the left coronary system, an aortogram in LAO projection is recommended. Conversely, for RCA grafts, an RAO projection should be adequate.

A careful review of native coronary angiograms may also provide clues regarding graft patency. For instance, if a bypassed native artery demonstrates competitive distal flow, the graft supplying that artery is likely patent. Conversely, if normal distal flow is seen in the bypassed native artery, without competitive filling, the graft is probably occluded.

Once properly engaged, each graft should be visualized in both the LAO and RAO projections using an injection technique similar to that employed for native coronaries. Usually, several views are needed to fully assess the graft ostium, body, and distal anastomosis. Additionally, the individual views that are best for evaluating each native coronary artery can be helpful in evaluating the distal anastomosis of the graft as well as the distal course of the native vessel.

Troubleshooting

Cannulating "Difficult" Grafts

SVG to LCX: This graft is usually the most cranially located graft within the ascending aorta. It is best engaged with a JR4 catheter while in the RAO projection, as are all grafts to the LCA system. Gentle clockwise rotation of the catheter at a location in the ascending aorta above the other SVGs will often successfully find the graft ostium. With all LCA grafts, the operator should strive to position the tip of the catheter so that it faces toward the right side of the aortic silhouette in the RAO view. Once engaged, the usual LAO and RAO views are subsequently obtained.

SVG to LAD and diagonal branches: The LAD graft is most commonly located above the ostium of the native LCA, and just beneath the ostium of the LCX graft described above. Again, with the JR4 catheter lying in the ascending aorta, clockwise rotation of the catheter usually locates the ostium of this graft. It often helps to rotate the catheter slightly above the suspected location of the ostium, as clockwise rotation usually brings the tip downward slightly. Occasionally, the JR4 catheter is unable to engage left coronary grafts, especially if there is an angulated takeoff from the aorta. A multipurpose or left coronary bypass (LCB) catheter can be useful in these settings.

SVG to RCA: This graft is commonly placed just above the native RCA ostium on the right side of the aorta. Engagement of this graft ostium is best facilitated with the camera in the LAO projection. Simply withdrawing the JR4 catheter from the RCA will often cannulate the graft ostium. If this fails, clockwise rotation of the catheter a few centimeters above the native RCA may bring the catheter into the correct plane. Sometimes, the takeoff of the RCA graft is at an acute angle from the aorta and is not easily cannulated with the JR4 catheter. A multipurpose catheter (usually a multipurpose B) can be helpful in such circumstances, as it has a more downward angle. Gentle clockwise rotation as this catheter is first withdrawn then advanced toward such a downwardly directed graft will usually place the catheter within the ostium. Right modified Amplatz, right coronary bypass (RCB), and 3-DRC catheters are other alternatives for cannulation of RCA grafts.

Internal Mammary Artery Grafts

Internal mammary artery (IMA) grafts are used routinely in coronary artery bypass surgery, as they provide superior patency rates compared to venous grafts in the long term. Left internal mammary artery (LIMA) graft patency has been reported to be 93% at 6 months and 90% at 10 years. When these arterial grafts do fail, **the culprit stenosis usually lies at the distal anastomosis or in the artery just beyond the anastomosis.**

In order to successfully cannulate the LIMA, the operator must understand the anatomy of the left subclavian artery and its branches. The LIMA is often anastomosed to the mid- or distal LAD, although it sometimes is grafted to diagonal branches or the left circumflex instead. It typically arises anteroinferiorly from the left subclavian artery, 1 to 3 cm beyond the vertebral artery (Figure 4-2).

Using the LAO projection, the JR4 catheter is positioned in the aortic arch just proximal to the origin of the left subclavian artery. The catheter is

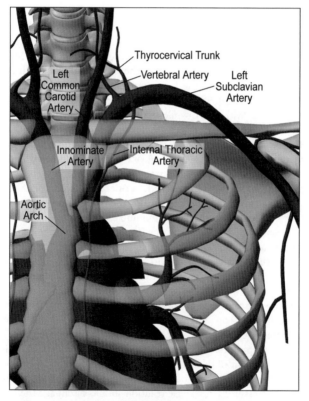

Figure **4-2** **This schematic depicts the typical anatomy of the left subclavian artery and its most proximal branches.** Note that the internal mammary (thoracic) artery (IMA) arises anteroinferiorly. When evaluating a patient with ischemia in the IMA distribution, it is important to rule out the possibility of subclavian or innominate stenosis proximal to the IMA origin.

then slowly pulled back as gentle counterclockwise rotation is applied, thereby moving the tip of the catheter superiorly into the origin of the left subclavian artery. An alternative technique for subclavian artery cannulation involves extending the tip of the JR4 catheter just past the left subclavian origin, then rotating the catheter clockwise to engage the artery. An angiogram of this artery in the posteroanterior (PA) projection enables the operator to locate the ostium of the LIMA and exclude a significant subclavian stenosis that could be indirectly causing myocardial ischemia by impairing flow down the LIMA. When the subclavian artery is tortuous, the origin of the LIMA is often better demonstrated in the RAO projection.

A 0.035-in guidewire (either the J-tipped wire or a Wholey wire) is then advanced gently through the catheter into the subclavian artery and out into the axillary artery, well beyond the origin of the LIMA. The catheter should then be advanced over the wire to a point about halfway between the sternum and the left shoulder. The guidewire is removed and the catheter is flushed vigorously. In order to engage the LIMA, the catheter is slowly withdrawn while simultaneously applying gentle counterclockwise rotation so that the catheter tip faces anteriorly. Because the LIMA often arises from the subclavian artery at a 90° angle, a catheter with a sharper curve, such as the IMA or 5-Fr. special IMA catheter, may be necessary to cannulate the ostium.

Small test injections can be used to orient the operator. **Nonionic contrast is advisable when injecting the subclavian and internal mammary arteries** in order to minimize the risk of hyperosmolar neurotoxicity, as well as to reduce the burning discomfort to the patient. Having the patient turn his/her head to the left or right can help engage the graft by slightly changing the orientation of the catheter.

Once the catheter nears the ostium of the mammary graft, the tip may "jump" into the ostium. One has to be extremely cautious when manipulating the catheter near or within the LIMA, as this vessel is especially delicate and prone to dissection (see Figure 3-7). For this reason, fine movements are advisable whenever attempting to engage the LIMA. If pressure damping does occur, the catheter tip should be quickly and carefully rotated out of the artery by rotating the catheter in an opposite direction. For example, if pullback and counterclockwise rotation resulted in a dampen pressure, a clockwise rotation should disengage the catheter from this position. In general, the catheter should never be advanced forward without a wire.

Once engaged, the LIMA graft is injected in at least two projections, paying special attention to the distal anastomotic site. Forceful injections are discouraged. Straight RAO and LAO projections are the most commonly employed. Cranial angulation can be added to either projection to better visualize the distal aspect of the LAD. A cross-table lateral view is sometimes helpful to gain an additional view of the anastomotic site.

If the LIMA cannot be selectively engaged, a subselective view can be obtained. In this instance, the catheter should be positioned as close as possible to the LIMA ostium. A blood pressure cuff inflated on the left arm will help direct contrast flow preferentially down the LIMA instead of distally into the brachial artery.

Selective visualization of the right internal mammary artery (RIMA) is similar to that of the LIMA above, but often is more difficult. A JR4 or IMA catheter (there is no specific RIMA catheter) is advanced into the proximal aortic arch past the origin of the innominate artery. Counterclockwise rotation will bring the tip of the catheter into the origin of the innominate artery, and a guidewire can subsequently be advanced through the catheter down the right subclavian artery, taking great care to avoid the right common carotid artery. The catheter is then advanced over the wire just as in LIMA catheterization. The difference in cannulating the RIMA is that upon pulling back the catheter, slow clockwise rotation is applied to bring the tip anteriorly to engage the RIMA ostium. When it is impossible to cannulate the RIMA with this technique, the operator may elect to configure a JR4 or IMA catheter with a concave secondary curve proximal to the primary curve in order to improve engagement of the RIMA ostium.

The RIMA (and occasionally even the LIMA) is often used as a "free" graft, with its proximal anastomosis in the ascending aorta. In this case, the procedure for cannulating the graft is the same as that for SVGs.

Radial Artery Grafts

On occasion, the angiographer may encounter a radial artery graft. Data suggest that short-term patency of radial artery grafts is comparable to that of SVGs. Long-term patency rates appear to be reasonable for radial artery grafts, with one study showing 92% patency at 5 to 7 years. Radial artery grafts are often placed in similar locations as SVGs, and they are cannulated in much the same way. Angiographically, these grafts have a smaller caliber and smoother appearance than their SVG counterparts.

Gastroepiploic Artery Grafts

The gastroepiploic artery (Figure 4-3) is a branch of the gastroduodenal artery, which originates from the common hepatic artery of the celiac trunk. It is seldom used but when it is employed as a conduit, it usually serves as an in situ graft to a vessel along the inferior surface of

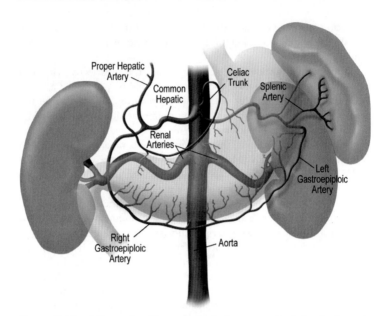

Figure **4-3** **Schematic diagram depicting normal abdominal aorta anatomy.** Note that the gastroepiploic artery is a branch of the common hepatic artery, which originates from the celiac trunk. The celiac trunk is typically located along the anterior aorta just proximal to the twelfth thoracic vertebra.

the heart, such as the posterior descending artery. The graft is usually cannulated with the use of a standard visceral catheter, such as the Cobra catheter. Subselective artery cannulation may erroneously lead to the conclusion that the graft is occluded, so it is important to selectively engage the artery.

Acknowledgments

The author would like to gratefully acknowledge the contributions of Christopher Merritt, MD, and Frederick A. Heupler, Jr, MD, to the first edition of this manuscript.

Suggested Reading

Isshiki T, Yamaguchi T, Nakamura T, et al. Postoperative angiographic evaluation of gastroepiploic artery grafts. *Cathet Cardiovasc Diagn*. 1990;21:233–228.

Peterson KL, Nicod P. *Cardiac Catheterization: Methods, Diagnosis, and Therapy.* 1st ed. Philadelphia: W.B. Saunders Co.; 1997:165–167.

Sabik JF III, Blackstone EH, Gillinov AM, et al. Occurrence and risk factors for reintervention after coronary artery bypass grafting. *Circulation*. 2006;114 (1 suppl):454–460.

Sabik JF III, Lytle BW, Blackstone EH, et al. Comparison of saphenous vein and internal thoracic artery graft patency by coronary system. *Ann Thorac Surg*. 2005;79(2):544–551.

Tatoulis J, Royse AG, Buxton BF, et al. The radial artery in coronary surgery: a 5-year experience—clinical and angiographic results. *Ann Thorac Surg*. 2002;73(1):143–147.

Tatoulis J, Buxton BF, Fuller JA. Patencies of 2127 arterial to coronary conduits over 15 years. *Ann Thorac Surg*. 2004;77(1):93–101.

Tatoulis J, Buxton BF, Fuller JA, et al. Long-term patency of 1108 radial arterial-coronary angiograms over 10 years. *Ann Thorac Surg*. 2009;88(1):23–29.

CHAPTER 5

Left Ventriculography and Aortography

Mateen Akhtar and Frederick A. Heupler, Jr.

Left ventriculography provides important anatomic and functional information that supplements coronary angiography. Left ventriculography allows assessment of left ventricular systolic function, degree of mitral regurgitation, and the presence/location of wall motion abnormality or ventricular septal defect (Table 5-1). Ventriculography should not be performed when a patient is hemodynamically unstable. Additional contraindications are listed in Table 5-2.

Preparation

Single-plane ventriculography is performed in most catheterization laboratories. Some operators prefer biplane ventriculography since it can provide more information about ventricular anatomy and function. Biplane ventriculography has limitations such as costly angiographic equipment, additional radiation exposure to both operator and patient, and longer angiographic setup time.

The Medrad powered flow injector is connected to extension tubing and loaded with contrast. During this process, air bubbles should be purged from the injector. Once appropriate pressure measurements have been obtained, the pigtail catheter is connected to extension tubing from the power injector via a blood-contrast interface to minimize the risk of air embolism with left ventriculography. Usually the left ventricular cavity is adequately visualized with 30 to 50 mL of contrast.

Table 5-1	Left Ventriculography: Indications

Assess global left ventricular systolic function and regional wall motion
Assess severity of mitral regurgitation
Identify and assess muscular and membranous ventricular septal defects

Table **5-2**	Left Ventriculography: Contraindications

Critical left main disease
Critical aortic stenosis
Fresh intracardiac thrombus[a]
Contrast media reaction
Tilting-disc aortic prosthesis
Decompensated heart failure and/or renal failure

[a]Because sessile thrombi more than 6 months old have a lower risk of dislodgement, some operators will proceed with ventriculography in this circumstance.

The parameters listed in Table 5-3 can serve as a baseline when deciding on the rate and volume of contrast injection. Certain patient characteristics and clinical settings will influence these settings. For instance, higher volumes of contrast dye (i.e., 50–60 mL) may be necessary to completely opacify the left atrium in patients with severe mitral regurgitation. Higher rates of contrast injection may be necessary in patients with increased cardiac output or dilated left ventricular cavity. Conversely, patients with smaller ventricular cavities such as elderly females or those with hypertensive heart disease may need only 30 to 36 mL of contrast dye for adequate imaging. **All patients with hemodynamically significant valvular disease, left ventricular dysfunction, or elevated left ventricular end-diastolic pressure (LVEDP) should receive nonionic contrast for ventriculography.**

Entering the Ventricle

The catheter most commonly used for ventriculography is an angled pigtail catheter. The distal segment of this catheter should be angled 145° to 155° in order to facilitate passage into the left ventricle while simultaneously preventing the endhole from contacting the endocardium, thereby reducing the risk of endocardial staining. The multiple side holes help dissipate the pressure of rapid power contrast injection and prevent excessive catheter movement.

Table **5-3**	Standard Settings for Left Ventriculography
Rate of rise	0–0.4 sec
Rate of injection	10–15 mL/sec
Volume of injection	30–40 cc
Maximum pressure	600–700 psi

The pigtail catheter is advanced over a 0.035-in J-tipped wire to a position in the ascending aorta just superior to the aortic valve. The tip should be pointed toward the orifice of the valve and the catheter rotated so that the pigtail loop resembles a "6." In this position, gently advancing the catheter will usually push it across the valve orifice and into the ventricle.

Occasionally, the pigtail catheter will prolapse into the ventricle while the pigtail remains in the ascending aorta. Slowly advancing the guidewire through the terminal portion of the catheter should provide enough additional support to allow entry into the ventricle. Once in the ventricle, the tip of the pigtail should be positioned in the midcavity avoiding contact with the papillary muscles and mitral valve (Figure 5-1).

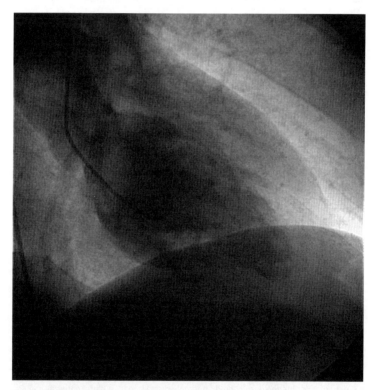

Figure **5-1**   **30° RAO ventriculogram demonstrating ideal placement of the pigtail catheter in the ventricular midcavity.** The most common reasons for ectopy during ventriculography are contact of the catheter with either the apex or the septum. Gentle counterclockwise rotation and/or pullback of the catheter should eliminate the ectopy.

Troubleshooting

Ventricular Ectopy

If the pigtail catheter irritates the apex, the risk of ventricular ectopy rises significantly. Gentle counterclockwise rotation and pullback should separate the catheter from the septal and apical walls and the ectopy will usually resolve.

Entrapment in Mitral Valve Apparatus

Occasionally, the catheter tip may become trapped within the mitral valve apparatus. If ventriculography is performed under these circumstances, transient but significant mitral regurgitation may develop. Gentle clockwise rotation should dislodge the catheter from the apparatus and place it in the center of the ventricle. If not, the catheter can be withdrawn from the ventricle and ventricular entry reattempted.

Once the catheter is stabilized within the left ventricle, it is connected to the pressure manifold, flushed, and used to record intraventricular pressures. Systolic pressure is typically recorded on a 200-mm Hg scale, while LVEDP is best appreciated on a 40-mm Hg scale. **Markedly elevated LVEDP (>30 mm Hg) usually precludes left ventriculography.** Administration of sublingual or intravenous nitroglycerin may reduce LVEDP to a more acceptable level.

In patients with compromised left ventricular systolic function, elevated LVEDP, or reduced creatinine clearance, a hand-injection left ventriculogram using digital subtraction angiography (DSA) may be preferred since

Troubleshooting

Crossing a Stenotic Aortic Valve

Crossing a stenotic aortic valve requires patience, experience, and a bit of luck. This task can be accomplished with a variety of catheters and wires depending on operator preference, experience, and patient anatomy. Some operators prefer a brief cine run of aortic valve opening and closing in right anterior oblique (RAO) and left anterior oblique (LAO) projections in order to identify the angle and plane of the aortic valve orifice prior to crossing it.

Due to the inherent thrombogenicity of guidewires, some operators advise administering 5,000 units of intravenous unfractionated heparin before attempting to cross a stenotic aortic valve. In addition, following every 3 minutes of unsuccessful wire manipulation, the wire should be removed and wiped, and the catheter should be flushed vigorously to prevent thrombus formation. Excessive force should never be used to pass the wire into the left ventricle. Common techniques for crossing a stenotic aortic valve are reviewed below.

Wire Selection

The most common wires utilized to cross a severely stenotic aortic valve are a straight-tipped wire (0.035 or 0.038) or a Rosen exchange J-tipped wire. The Rosen wire is a J-tipped wire with a J-curve that is narrower (5 mm diameter) than the usual J-tip (10 mm diameter). The advantage of the Rosen wire is that the J-tip eliminates the risk of left ventricular perforation, but it may be more difficult to pass across a very severely stenotic valve. The advantage of a straight-tipped wire is that it will cross virtually any stenotic aortic valve, but the straight tip can perforate the left ventricle. The safest procedure is to initially attempt to cross the valve with the Rosen wire, which can be accomplished in more than 90% of cases.

Catheter Selection

Common catheters utilized to cross the aortic valve are the pigtail, Amplatz left coronary, Feldman, Judkins right coronary, and multipurpose catheters. The Amplatz and Feldman catheters are preferred if the aorta is dilated. The length of the secondary curve of these catheters should be adjusted proportionally to the diameter of the aorta. The Judkins right coronary and multipurpose catheters are preferred when the aortic root is narrow.

Technique

Once the selected catheter is positioned in the ascending aorta, the guidewire is cautiously advanced through the endhole of the catheter in an attempt to cross the valve orifice. Carefully advancing and rotating the catheter simultaneously should eventually direct the wire across the aortic valve. The tip of the wire should be directed anteriorly and to the patient's left. Generally, it is easier to cross the valve in the RAO projection. The angiographer should only attempt to advance the wire across the valve during systole. Altering the amount of wire protruding from the pigtail catheter may help direct the wire. For instance, more wire protruding from the pigtail catheter directs the wire toward the right coronary sinus, whereas less wire protruding directs the wire to the left coronary sinus.

Crossing a Prosthetic Aortic Valve

Crossing a prosthetic stenotic aortic valve is typically not clinically necessary but may be considered when echocardiography provides suboptimal image quality, when echocardiographic and clinical findings do not correlate, or when there is severe left ventricular dysfunction with low cardiac output. It is absolutely contraindicated to cross a tilting-disc aortic valve prosthesis (St. Jude, Medtronic-Hall, Bjork-Shiley). Attempts at catheter or wire passage across these prostheses can result in entrapment and/or disc dislodgement. Bioprosthetic porcine and pericardial valves may be crossed. In theory, Starr–Edwards prosthetic valves may also be crossed, but smaller sized catheters are usually necessary. **Avoid crossing a metal prosthesis unless absolutely necessary**.

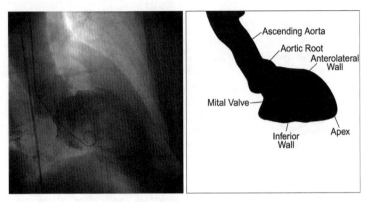

Figure **5-2**   Left ventriculogram in a 30° RAO view.

only 10 mL of contrast is needed. Patients should be instructed to cease respiration and avoid any motion during cine acquisition in order to minimize artifact.

Views

The most common views for left ventriculography are the 30° RAO and 60° LAO projections. The optimal magnification is a 9-in field because it allows for complete visualization of the entire left ventricle, including the mitral and aortic valves, without the need for panning.

30° RAO View: The 30° RAO view is particularly helpful because it projects the left ventricle off the spine, thus producing a higher quality picture (Figure 5-2). Positioning the wedge filter into the upper right hand corner improves image quality. The walls best visualized with the 30° RAO view include the anterior, apical, and inferior walls. Also, from this angle the mitral valve is seen in profile, allowing for evaluation of mitral valve disease. One limitation of this view is that it places the left atrium over the spine and descending aorta, thus impairing the operator's ability to evaluate the severity of mitral regurgitation. Adding steeper RAO angulation (45°) will help the operator quantify mitral regurgitation since this view positions the left atrium to the right of the spine.

60° LAO View: The 60° LAO view is most useful for functional assessment of the ventricular septum, lateral wall, and posterior walls (Figure 5-3).

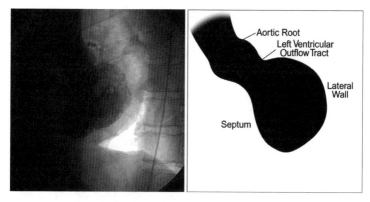

Figure **5-3**   Left ventriculogram in a 60° LAO view.

Also, the aortic valve is well visualized. Adding 25° of cranial angulation reduces any foreshortening of the ventricular septum and therefore is ideal for assessing the left ventricular outflow tract and for presence of a muscular ventricular septal defect. Cranial angulation also provides improved visualization of the left atrium because it positions the left atrium away from the spine, the left ventricle, and the descending aorta.

Left Lateral View (70° to 80°): A lateral view is particularly useful to assess for a membranous ventricular septal defect.

Analysis

Left Ventricular Systolic Function: In most laboratories, a qualitative assessment of left ventricular systolic function, mitral regurgitation severity, and regional wall motion is performed. When describing regional wall motion, the walls are commonly classified as either normal, hypokinetic, akinetic, or dyskinetic (Table 5-4). Once all the ventricular walls have

Table **5-4** Classification of Regional Wall Motion	
Classification	**Definition**
Hypokinesia	Reduction of inward motion during systole
Akinesia	Absence of inward motion during systole
Dyskinesia	Paradoxical outward motion during systole

Table **5-5**	Semiquantitative Assessment of LV Systolic Function
LV Systolic Function	**Ejection Fraction**
Normal	≥55–60%
Low normal	50%
Mildly impaired	40–49%
Moderately impaired	30–39%
Severely impaired	≤30%

been studied, an estimation of global left ventricular systolic function is made. This estimation is typically done semiquantitatively (Table 5-5). A quantitative assessment of left ventricular systolic function may be calculated by comparing end-systolic to end-diastolic left ventricular volume. However, these calculations are rarely done on a routine basis.

Valvular Anatomy and Function: During left ventriculography, both aortic and mitral valve function should be grossly assessed. Table 5-6 classifies degrees of mitral regurgitation. Leaflet mobility, thickening, and calcification can each be evaluated. Mitral annular calcification, if present, should be noted and quantified. Bicuspid aortic valves and mitral valve prolapse may also be observed.

Prosthetic Valves: The ideal angulation for either the RAO or LAO view places the annulus of the prosthesis perpendicular to the imaging plane. **The best angle for evaluating mitral valve function is an RAO**

Table **5-6**	Angiographic Assessment of Mitral Regurgitation
Grade	**Angiographic Appearance**
Mild (1+)	Faint LA opacification that clears with each beat does not opacify the entire LA
Moderate (2+)	Complete LA opacification after several beats Opacification intensity: LA $\ll$ LV
Moderately severe (3+)	Complete LA opacification Opacification intensity: LA = LV
Severe (4+)	Complete LA opacification after one beat Opacification intensity: LA $\gg$ LV Opacification of pulmonary veins

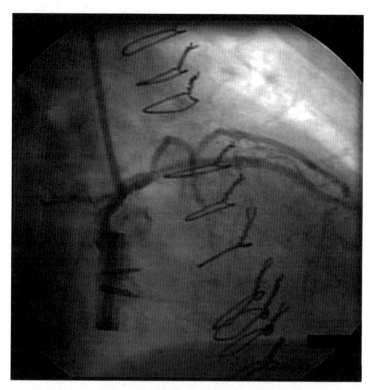

Figure **5-4** An RAO projection of a normally functioning bileaflet tilting-disc (St. Jude's) mitral valve prosthesis. (Courtesy of Mario Garcia, MD.)

view (Figure 5-4). The best angle for evaluating aortic valve function is an LAO view (Figure 5-5).

A complete fluoroscopic evaluation includes assessment of valvular motion and structural integrity. Some prosthetic valve companies, such as St. Jude's and Bjork-Shiley, publish what they consider to be normal parameters for opening and closing angles. These angles can be measured fluoroscopically to determine if a specific valve is functioning properly. However, the availability of multiplane transesophageal echocardiography (TEE) obviates the need for angiographic assessment of prosthetic valve function in most cases.

Complications

Potential complications of left ventriculography are listed in Table 5-7.

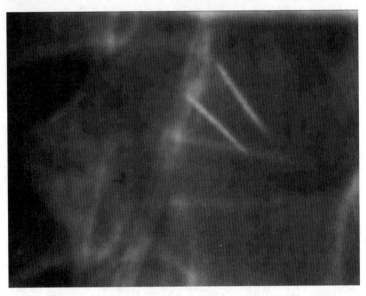

Figure **5-5** An LAO projection of a normally functioning bileaflet tilting-disc aortic valve prosthesis. (Courtesy of Mario Garcia, MD.)

Table **5-7**	Complications of Left Ventriculography
Complication	**Caveats**
Ventricular arrhythmias	Most common complication
	Sustained VT is an indication for immediate wire/catheter removal
Complete heart block	Complete heart block may occur due to trauma from the catheter as it enters the left ventricle or during ventriculography. Particular caution should be used in patients with baseline RBBB and left posterior hemiblock
Endocardial staining	Refers to accumulation of contrast within endocardium
	Larger stains may result in VT or VF
Air embolism	Potentially catastrophic complication which may result in CVA or MI
Cardiac tamponade	Catastrophic complication which occurs if ventricle is punctured during aggressive wire manipulation; rare with reported incidence of 0.3%

VT, ventricular tachycardia; VF, ventricular fibrillation; RBBB, right bundle branch block; CVA, cerebrovascular accident; MI, myocardial infarction.

Table **5-8**	Aortography: Common Indications and Contraindications

Indications

Assess severity of aortic regurgitation
Assess aneurysm size
Identify the location and extent of aortic dissection
Opacify difficult-to-find bypass grafts or anomalous coronary arteries
Localize coarctation of the aorta

Contraindications

Decompensated heart failure
Renal failure
Contrast media reaction

Aortography

Introduction: Aortography is not routinely performed during diagnostic cardiac catheterization. However, in certain circumstances (Table 5-8), aortography can be useful to better define aortic root anatomy (Table 5-9) and aortic valve function (Table 5-10).

Preparation: A 6-French pigtail catheter is most commonly employed because its multiple side holes reduce the risk for aortic dissection during power injection. The pigtail is advanced to a location just above the

Table **5-9**	Normal Aortic Anatomy

Location	Description
Aortic root or bulb	Formed by the three sinuses of Valsalva: right, left, and posterior
Ascending aorta	Measures 2.2–3.8 cm in normal adults
Aortic arch	Gives rise to the great vessels including the brachiocephalic, left common carotid, and left subclavian artery
Descending aorta	Continuation of aorta distal to left subclavian artery Typically measures ~2.5 cm Anatomic landmark used to distinguish type A from type B dissections

Table **5-10**	Angiographic Assessment of Aortic Insufficiency
Grade	**Angiographic Appearance**
Mild (1+)	Faint, incomplete LV opacification that clears with each beat
Moderate (2+)	Opacification of entire LV << aorta
Moderately severe (3+)	Progressive opacification of entire LV = aorta
Severe (4+)	Dense LV opacification after one beat >> aorta

sinotubular junction. Standard injection volume is 40 to 60 mL at a rate of 20 mL/sec.

Views: The most useful view is a 60° LAO view because both the aortic root anatomy and the severity of aortic insufficiency can be evaluated (Figure 5-6).

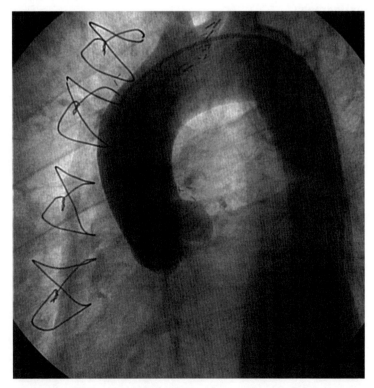

Figure **5-6**   60° LAO aortography demonstrating a normal aorta.

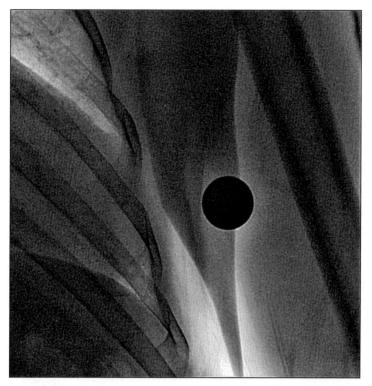

Figure **5-7**   An object with a predefined diameter may be placed in the fluoroscopic field and used as a reference when measuring aortic aneurysms, for instance.

Analysis: In order to measure aortic root dimensions, image acquisition of a radiopaque standard-sized object is used as a reference (Figure 5-7). The diameter of this object is measured during angiography and then used to calculate the diameter of the aortic root. Once an image of the object has been obtained, aortic root angiography must be performed using the same angulation and magnification.

Assessment of Aortic Dissection: Aortography may help identify the origin and proximal and/or distal extension of an aortic dissection (Figure 5-8). In addition, the severity of aortic regurgitation, the patency of the proximal coronary arteries, and location of an intimal flap may also be evaluated. It is important never to inject into the false lumen of an aortic dissection. **With advances in noninvasive imaging modalities such as**

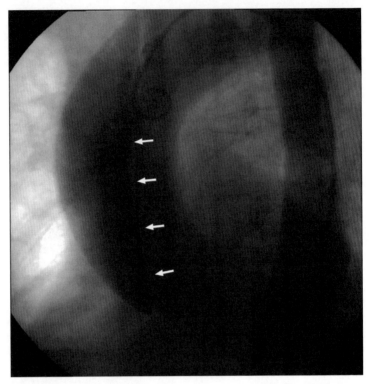

Figure **5-8** **An example of an ascending aortic dissection in LAO projection.** Note the "flap" visualized *(arrows).*

TEE, cardiac CT, and MRI, aortography is no longer the initial imaging modality of choice in the diagnosis of aortic dissection.

Locating Bypass Grafts: **Aortography is sometimes performed to help locate difficult-to-find bypass grafts.** It is important to remember, however, that lack of bypass graft opacification by aortography does not completely rule out the presence of patent grafts.

Coarctation of the Aorta: Aortic coarctation is best identified from a lateral view (Figure 5-9). Aortography determines the site of obstruction and extent of pre and/or poststenotic dilatation. A pressure gradient >20 mm Hg across the coarctation is considered to be hemodynamically significant, while a gradient >50 mm Hg warrants intervention.

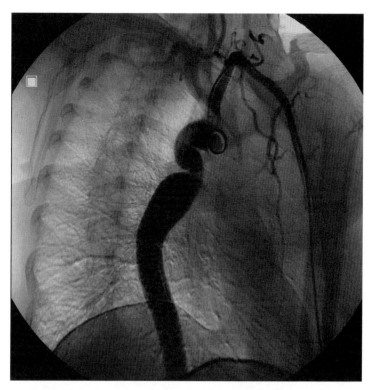

Figure **5-9**   Example of coarctation of the aorta in steep RAO projection.

Suggested Reading

Arciniegas JG, Soto B, Little WC, et al. Cineangiographs in the diagnosis of aortic dissection. *Am J Cardiol.* 1981;47:890–894.

Baltaxe HA. Imaging of the left ventricle in patients with ischemic heart disease: role of the contrast angiogram. *Cardiovasc Intervent Radiol.* 1982;5: 137–144.

Bhargava V, Warren S, Vieweg WVR, et al. Quantitation of left ventricular wall motion in normal subjects: comparison of various methods. *Cathet Cardiovasc Diagn.* 1980;6:7–16.

Chaitman BR, DeMots H, Bristow JD, et al. Objective and subjective analysis of left ventricular angiograms. *Circulation.* 1975;52:420–425.

Sanders C. Current role of conventional and digital aortography in the diagnosis of aortic disease. *J Thorac Imaging.* 1990;5:48–59.

CHAPTER 6

Cerebral and Peripheral Angiography

Inder M. Singh, Steven J. Filby,
and Mehdi H. Shishehbor

Noncoronary angiography, often generalized as "peripheral" angiography, has become an increasingly common part of the invasive cardiologist's repertoire. Prior to gaining a sound working knowledge of peripheral angiography, it is important to recognize several associated salient technical features. It is also prudent to have a sound knowledge of the key elements that distinguish peripheral from coronary angiography.

1. The diameter of the image intensifier used for peripheral angiography is 14 to 16 in compared to 9 in used in most cardiac catheterization laboratories. This provides a larger imaging window when viewing the aorta and lower extremities.
2. The frame rate for peripheral angiography is usually 2 to 3 frames per second compared to 15 to 30 frames per second for coronary angiography.
3. Digital subtraction angiography (DSA) is the preferred imaging modality for peripheral angiography. DSA literally subtracts the surrounding radio structures (such as bone) and shows only the contrast-filled arterial bed of interest. This technique greatly enhances image quality but requires the patient to be completely still (including temporary cessation of respiration or swallowing for carotid angiography) during image acquisition. The radiation exposure for DSA is significantly greater than standard cardiac cineangiography.
4. Trace subtract fluoroscopy or "road mapping" is frequently used instead of standard fluoroscopy during peripheral angiography. Like DSA, "road mapping" also enables visualization of contrast-filled vessels without the surrounding tissues or bone.
5. Arterial access for peripheral angiography may require retrograde common femoral artery (CFA) cannulation. However, depending on the nature of disease, antegrade CFA cannulation or brachial/radial

access may be required. **Prior to upper extremity access, an Allen test should be performed to confirm intact dual vascular supply of the hand.** Familiarity with the micropuncture system is essential for all physicians performing peripheral angiography.

6. Ionic contrast is not used for peripheral angiography as it has been associated with transient vision loss during cerebrovascular angiography and is extremely painful when used for limb angiography. A nonionic iso-osmolar agent such as iodixanol is the preferred contrast agent.

Similarities in the periprocedural evaluation of patients undergoing coronary or peripheral angiography are enumerated below.

1. Knowledge of presenting symptoms is essential for clinical and technical decision making.

2. Knowledge of comorbid medical conditions is important for performing the procedure safely.

3. Knowledge of angiography and prior revascularization in any vascular bed is imperative. **Reviewing noninvasive data from peripheral computed tomography and magnetic resonance angiography can be extremely helpful for planning access and strategy.** This becomes especially important in cases of complete occlusion and also in cases of prior bypass grafting. **It is also important to note the timing of bypass grafts, as direct cannulation of grafts less than 6 months old should be avoided when possible.**

4. A focused physical examination pre- and post-procedure is mandatory and should include access site examination and a full assessment of all relevant vascular beds proximally and distally for pulses, bruit, thrills, or presence of hematoma. Additionally, a pre- and postfocused neurologic examination should be performed for carotid and cerebral angiography.

5. Standard preangiography laboratory evaluation is necessary for patient safety.

6. Medications such as warfarin and metformin should be held prior to peripheral angiography in a manner similar to coronary angiography.

Cerebrovascular

Anatomy: The aortic arch is the major conduit that gives rise to the entire cerebrovascular system (Figure 6-1). The aortic arch is classified as type 1, 2, or 3 based on plane and angle of takeoff of its major branches. As part of the aging process, the aortic arch can remodel from type 1 (horizontal plane) to type 3 (C-shaped plane) as the arch sinks into the thoracic cavity. Traditionally, the arterial branches arise off the arch in

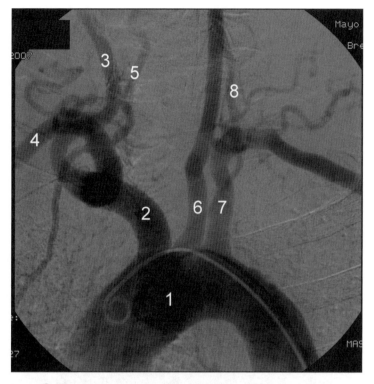

Figure **6-1** **Aortic arch and great vessels.** 1: aortic arch; 2: innominate; 3: right common carotid; 4: right subclavian; 5: right vertebral; 6: left common carotid; 7: left subclavian; 8: left vertebral.

the following order: (1) innominate artery, (2) left common carotid artery (CCA), and (3) left subclavian artery (SCA). The innominate bifurcates into the right SCA and the right CCA. The right and left SCA give rise to their respective vertebral arteries. A more detailed description of the SCA and its branches is presented in the "Upper Extremity/ Thorax" section later in this chapter.

The right CCA usually arises from the bifurcation of the innominate artery (Figure 6-1). Occasionally, the right CCA may arise independently from the aortic arch. Rarely, the right and left CCA may arise as a common carotid trunk from the arch. The left CCA has significant variation in its anatomy. In 75% of individuals, it is the second great vessel arising from the aortic arch, posterior to the innominate. In the remaining cases, the origin of the left CCA is via a shared origin with the innominate off the aortic arch or as a branch off the innominate proper (also known as a "bovine arch"). Although there is significant variation, the CCA typically bifurcates into the external carotid artery (ECA) and the internal carotid artery (ICA), at the upper border of the thyroid cartilage (Figure 6-2). The CCA usually does not give off any significant branches until it bifurcates into the ICA and ECA.

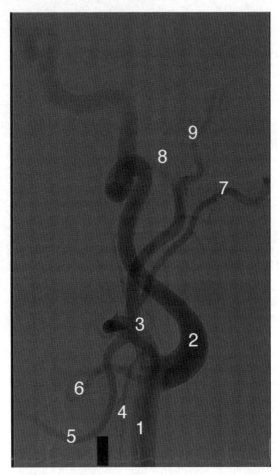

Figure **6-2** **Left carotid.** 1: common carotid; 2: internal carotid; 3: external carotid; 4: superior thyroid; 5: facial; 6: lingual; 7: occipital; 8: maxillary; 9: superficial temporal. The ascending pharyngeal and posterior auricular branches of the external carotid are not clearly appreciated.

The ECA is readily recognized due to its eight extracranial branches. These arterial branches arise in the following order—superior thyroid, ascending pharyngeal, lingual, occipital, facial, posterior auricular, maxillary, and superficial temporal (Figure 6-2).

The ICA is recognized by the bulbous carotid sinus at its origin. This region houses the mechano- and chrono-regulatory receptors for the body. Conventionally, the ICA is divided into four segments—cervical, petrosal, cavernous, and supraclinoid (sometimes also referred to as subarachnoid).

1. Cervical segment: The segment between the CCA bifurcation and the petrous bone. This segment does not give off any arterial branches. The ostial and proximal portions of this segment are often involved in carotid atherosclerotic disease.
2. Petrosal segment: The segment that courses through the petrous bone to the cavernous sinus. This segment has the shape of an inverted hockey stick. This segment also does not give off any arterial branches.
3. Cavernous segment: The segment that courses through the cavernous sinus giving off the meningiohypophyseal and the inferior cavernous sinus arterial branch.
4. Supraclinoid segment: The segment begins after the ICA exits the cavernous sinus. Several key branches that originate from this segment include the ophthalmic, posterior communicating, and anterior choroidal. The ICA terminates after this segment in the anterior and middle cerebral artery. Thus, the main area of the brain supplied by the anterior and middle cerebral arteries is referred to as the carotid territory. The classical finding of amaurosis fugax results from ophthalmic artery ischemia.

Other important extracranial vessels include the bilateral vertebral arteries that anastamose at the base of the pons to give rise to a single basilar artery, which lies intracranially. The largest branches of the vertebral arteries are the bilateral posterior inferior cerebellar arteries, while the basilar artery gives off bilateral anterior inferior cerebellar arteries, superior cerebellar arteries, and the posterior cerebral arteries. These arteries form the posterior circulation of the brain including the cerebellar blood supply. Usually, the left vertebral circulation is dominant and provides the majority of the arterial supply to this region.

The intracranial circulation is formed by the anterior cerebral artery, anterior communicating artery, middle cerebral artery, posterior cerebral artery, and posterior communicating artery (Figure 6-3). The circle of Willis is formed by these vessels but a "normal ring" is found only in 50% of individuals. Description of the anatomic variations is beyond the scope of this text.

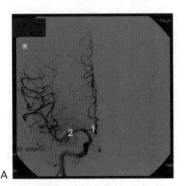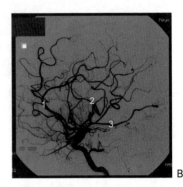

A   B

Figure **6-3**   **A) Right intracranial circulation (anteroposterior projection).** 1: anterior cerebral; 2: middle cerebral. **B) Right intracranial circulation (lateral projection).** 1: anterior cerebral; 2: middle cerebral; 3: posterior cerebral.

Angiography: Aortic arch angiography is the recommended first step prior to selective angiography of the cerebrovascular system (Figure 6-1). This allows for assessment of arch type, detection of anomalous vessel origin or takeoff, and estimation of proximal vessel atherosclerosis and tortuosity. Arch angiography is generally performed with a power contrast injection (20 mL per second for 40 mL total) using a standard multihole pigtail catheter approximately 40° left anterior oblique (LAO). For arch angiography, the patient should be asked to turn his or her head to the right in an extended position.

Carotid angiography and catheter selection is determined by aortic arch type. In type 1 and most type 2 arches, the carotids can be successfully engaged using a JR4 diagnostic catheter. For type 2 arches with bovine left CCA origin or type 3 arches, a Vitek catheter is usually required. **A heparin bolus of 2,000 to 3,000 units should be administered prior to selective angiography of the cerebrovascular system.** Before engaging the great vessels, the arch angiogram should be used as a reference view on the monitor. For the right CCA, the innominate is first engaged; and the right anterior oblique (RAO) projection is used to separate the ostia of the right-sided SCA and CCA. In most cases, the diagnostic catheter can be carefully advanced to engage the right CCA. If there is any difficulty in engaging the ostium of the right CCA, a soft wire such as a Wholey or a stiff-angled Glidewire can be used to advance the catheter to the proximal portion of the CCA. The left CCA is selectively engaged directly off the aortic arch. In general, all catheter advancements should be performed over a wire.

The standard views to assess for carotid disease are ipsilateral oblique views between 30° and 45° and the left lateral view to

Troubleshooting

1. Air and clot embolization: Embolization of either air or clots in the cerebral vasculature can lead to catastrophic consequences. Thus, a meticulous technique with regular checks for air or clots and frequent flushing of catheters with heparanized saline is essential. Catheter exchanges should be kept to the minimum during cerebrovascular angiography. When exchanges are performed, extreme care should be taken to wipe the wire of any clots and to flush catheter and access sheath.
2. Ostial stenosis of the vertebral artery: When the vertebral artery ostium is diseased, direct engagement with a diagnostic catheter is not recommended as this may cause embolization of the ostial plaque and posterior territory infarct. Thus, in situations of verterbral ostial disease, a nonselective angiogram should be obtained instead as described above.

initially define the carotid bifurcation. The angle of mandible serves as a useful landmark for carotid bifurcation. Since the proximal ICA lies posterior and medial to the ECA, lateral and posteroanterior (PA) views may also be necessary to define the anatomy (Figure 6-2).

Selective engagement of the vertebrals can often be achieved using a JR4 catheter or a Headhunter catheter using the same technique as with the carotids. However, nonselective angiography of the vertebrals is routinely performed with the tip of the diagnostic catheter close to but not directly engaged with the ostia. An ipsilateral arm blood pressure cuff is inflated to maximize visualization during nonselective angiograms. A single ipsilateral oblique view is adequate in most cases.

The anterior and middle cerebral circulation is best visualized in a shallow PA view at 15° to 30° (Figure 6-3). Positioning the petrous bone at the base of the orbit in this projection serves as a useful landmark. The intracranial posterior circulation is best seen in a steep PA view at 40° (Figure 6-3). Lateral views are also frequently used for all three intracranial circulations.

Upper Extremity

Anatomy: The right SCA arises from the bifurcation of the innominate, whereas the left SCA arises as the third and final branch off the aortic arch (Figures 6-1 and 6-4). In 0.5% percent of cases, the right SCA arises as the last branch of the descending thoracic aorta. In its proximal segment, the SCA first gives off the vertebral artery followed by the internal mammary artery (IMA), the latter of which supplies the anterior chest wall (Figure 6-4). In 1% to 5% of individuals, the left vertebral artery arises directly from aortic arch. The thyrocervical and costocervical trunks arise from the midsegment of SCA and give

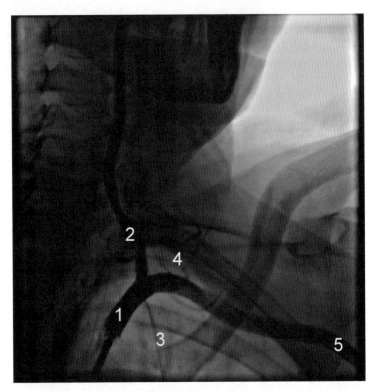

Figure **6-4**   **Left upper extremity.** 1: subclavian; 2: vertebral; 3: internal mammary; 4: thyrocervical trunk; 5: axillary.

branches to the thyroid gland, cervical muscles, ribs, and the scapular region (Figure 6-4).

At the lateral margin of the first rib, the SCA becomes the axillary artery (Figure 6-4). The axillary artery becomes the brachial artery at the neck of the humeral bone. At the neck of the radius bone, the brachial artery divides into the radial and ulnar arteries. Occasionally, the radial artery can originate from the axillary artery (1–3%) or higher in the course of the brachial artery (15–20%). The ulnar artery forms the superficial palmar arch and the radial artery forms the deep palmar arch, although anatomic variations are common (Figure 6-5).

Angiography: Aortic arch angiography is the recommended first step prior to selective angiography for reasons detailed earlier in this chapter (Figure 6-1). Selective angiography of the innominate and the left SCA

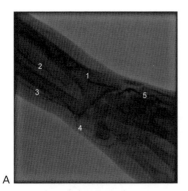 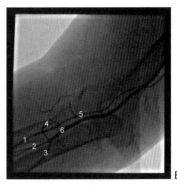

A   B

Figure **6-5**   **A) Left upper extremity.** 1: radial; 2: interosseous; 3: ulnar; 4: superficial palmar arch; 5: deep palmar arch. **B) Left upper extremity.** 1: radial; 2: interosseous; 3: ulnar; 4: radial loop; 5: accessory radial; 6: brachial.

can usually be accomplished with the standard 5-Fr. JR4 diagnostic catheter. For more difficult arches, alternative catheters such as Vitek, Simmons, or Headhunter may be necessary. Angiography of the SCA is done with the arm adducted in the neutral position using 5 to 10 mL injections under DSA.

Innominate artery angiography is done in the RAO projection which separates the bifurcation of the right CCA and ostium of the right-sided SCA. Orthogonal oblique projections are used to demonstrate the initial branches of the SCA (Figure 6-4). The right vertebral and right IMA are visualized in the RAO view, while the left vertebral and left IMA are best evaluated in the LAO projection.

Upper extremity angiography is done by advancing the diagnostic catheter, over a Wholey or angled Glidewire, into the distal SCA for views of the axillary or brachial anatomy and into the distal brachial artery for radial or ulnar angiography. Upper extremity angiography is done in the PA projection, but appropriate limb positioning is important (Figure 6-5). The axillary artery is imaged with the arm in the neutral position, while the brachial artery is best visualized with the arm abducted and the forearm supine (on an arm board). For the forearm and hand arteries, the forearm should be supine on the arm board with the palm facing up, the thumb abducted, and the fingers splayed.

Mesenteric and Renal

Anatomy: The first major branch of the abdominal aorta is the celiac trunk which arises at the level of the T12 vertebrae (Figure 6-6). The celiac trunk divides into the left gastric, common hepatic, and splenic

Troubleshooting

1. Access issues: Arterial access can be via the ipsilateral brachial or radial if there is severe peripheral and aortic disease, type 3 arch, severe subclavian tortuosity, or occlusion of the SCA.
2. Patients with thoracic outlet syndrome causing arterial compression: Angiography is first performed with the arm in a neutral adducted position under PA projection and then repeated with the arm abducted at the shoulder, externally rotated and retroverted, similar to a throwing position. Additional positions may be necessary depending on the patient's symptoms.
3. Spasm of the brachial or arm arteries: A cocktail of vasodilators such as nitroglycerine (200–400 μg) and verapamil (500–1000 μg) in multiple doses should be liberally used to prevent or relieve spasm of the upper extremity vessels and to improve visualization of the distal vessels.
4. Poor visualization of the digital vessels: Wrap the hand with a warm cloth to promote vasodilation and improve visualization.
5. Image quality is compromised by motion artifact: If despite educating the patient, motion artifact corrupts the image quality, then the patient's hand and fingers should be taped to an armboard to maintain stability.

arteries and, in so doing, supplies the stomach, liver, and parts of the esophagus, spleen, duodenum, and pancreas. The superior mesenteric artery (SMA) arises inferior to the celiac trunk, at the level of the L1 vertebrae. The SMA courses downward to supply the lower aspect of the duodenum and the pancreas by branching into the inferior pancreatico-duodenal, middle colic, right colic, ileocolic, and intestinal arteries. The middle colic, right colic, and ileocecal branches anastamose with the left colic artery (given off of the inferior mesenteric artery [IMA]) to form the marginal artery (artery of Drummond). The IMA arises below the renal arteries at approximately the L3 level and courses inferiorly from the anterior aorta giving off the left colic artery and sigmoid branches before terminating in the superior rectal artery.

The renal arteries generally arise from the lateral aspect of the descending aorta at the level between the L1 and L2 vertebrae (Figure 6-7). Although the right kidney sits lower in the abdomen than the left, the right renal artery typically originates slightly higher than the left. And while the right renal artery usually may have a slight anterior takeoff, the origin of both renal arteries from the lateral aspect of the aorta is variable. The main renal artery typically continues for several millimeters before dividing into segmental branches which subsequently terminate as interlobular and arcuate branches within the renal cortex and medulla. The presence of accessory renal arteries is not uncommon. These acces-

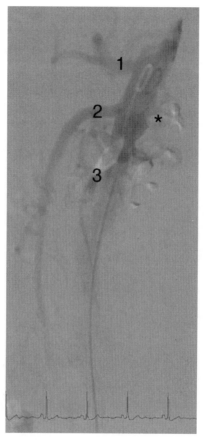

Figure **6-6**   **Mesenteric.** 1: celiac; 2: superior mesenteric; 3: inferior mesenteric. *Calcified and thrombosed aortic aneurysm.

sory vessels usually arise below the main renal artery and can be of smaller or equal caliber compared to the parent vessel. Another variant is the early bifurcation of the main vessel into segmental vessels.

Angiography: Abdominal angiography is routinely performed, in the PA projection, using a multihole pigtail or an Omni Flush catheter placed at the T12 vertebrae. This is typically performed prior to selective renal or mesenteric angiography. It allows for evaluation of the aortic calcification and aortic aneurysmal dilation in the region of the renal arteries along with examination of the renal ostia and presence of

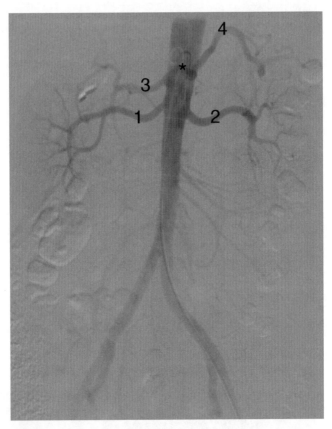

Figure **6-7   Renal and mesenteric.** 1: right renal; 2: left renal; 3: common hepatic; 4: splenic. *The origin of the celiac trunk is "end on" and thus not seen. The left gastric branch of the celiac trunk is also not clearly appreciated.

anatomic anomalies. **For visualization of the mesenteric vessels, a lateral view abdominal aortogram best demonstrates the origins of the mesenteric vessels since these arise anteriorly** (Figure 6-6).

For selective mesenteric and renal angiography, 4-Fr. to 6-Fr. catheters are typically used with a femoral access site. A JR4, internal mammary (IMA), or left coronary bypass (LCB) are most often used to selectively cannulate the SMA, IMA, and celiac trunk. However, catheters with a reverse angle such as the SoS catheter can also be used to engage these vessels. Alternatively, if a brachial or radial access is used, the mesenteric arteries can also be cannulated with a multipurpose or JR4 catheter.

Troubleshooting

1. Difficulty visualizing renal ostia: Renal artery ostial disease may be missed by standard angiography. Thus, if clinical suspicion of RAS is high, extreme oblique projections with added cranial or caudal angulation may be needed to better lay out the renal ostia. Intravascular ultrasound (IVUS) can also be used for better visualization of the renal arteries and to determine the presence of renal artery ostial disease. Damping of the catheter upon engagement may indicate a significant ostial lesion.
2. Patients with severe renal insufficiency and suboptimal or equivocal noninvasive studies: Carbon dioxide imaging can be used instead of iso-osmolar contrast imaging. Gadolinium has been associated with nephrogenic systemic fibrosis in patients with advanced renal failure and thus is also not used.

The renal arteries can be engaged with a JR4, internal mammary (IMA), or an SoS catheter. In cases of severe aortoiliac tortuosity, alternative catheters such as the C2 Cobra catheter may be necessary.

Selective angiography of the celiac trunk is usually performed in a PA projection or slight RAO or LAO angulation. The SMA and IMA have a downward course toward the pelvis. Selective SMA and IMA angiography is best performed in a lateral or steep LAO projection. A 15° to 30° LAO oblique view enables good visualization of the renal ostia and proximal segment; and slight cranial or caudal angulation is sometimes necessary for optimal visualization. It is important not only to visualize the renal ostia but also to determine the amount of associated aortic calcification in relation to the ostia. **A major pattern to recognize is the classic "beads on a string" appearance of fibromuscular dysplasia that occurs most commonly in young women and accounts for 10% of cases with renal artery stenosis (RAS).** Finally, when performing renal angiography, the field of view should be large enough to visualize the contrast in the renal cortex (Figure 6-7). Such nephrographic imaging is important to gain insight into renal size and regional function. This is especially important in individuals with suboptimal or equivocal noninvasive studies.

Lower Extremity

Anatomy: The descending aorta divides into the bilateral common iliac arteries at the level of L3–L4 (Figure 6-8). The common iliac artery (CIA) further divides into the external iliac and internal iliac arteries at the pelvic inlet anterior to the sacroiliac joint. The internal iliac artery (IIA) and its branches supply the pelvic organs and gluteal region. The external iliac

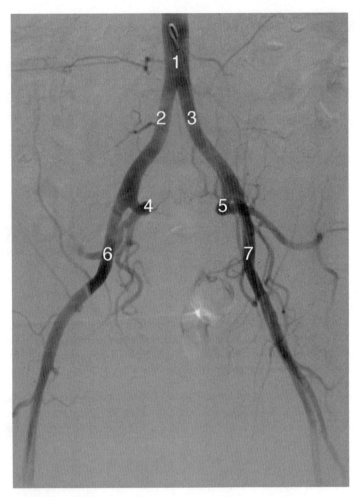

Figure **6-8   Aortoiliac system.** 1: aortic bifurcation; 2: right common iliac; 3: left common iliac; 4: right internal iliac; 5: left internal iliac; 6: right external iliac; 7: left external iliac.

artery (EIA) runs along the medial border of the psoas muscle and passes under the iliac ligament to become the CFA.

The CFA lies midway between the anterior superior iliac spine and the symphysis pubis (Figure 6-9). It transitions to the superficial femoral artery (SFA) at the inferior margin of the femoral head. The SFA runs medially and anteriorly, passing through the femoral triangle proximally and the adductor canal in the mid-thigh. The SFA rarely gives off

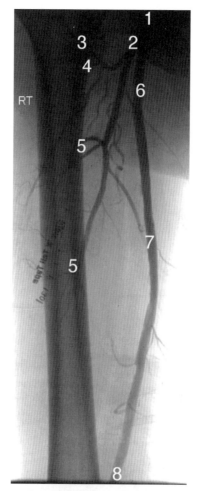

Figure **6-9** **Right femoral system.** 1: common femoral; 2: profunda femoris; 3: medial circumflex; 4: lateral circumflex; 5: perforating branches; 6: superficial femoral in the femoral triangle; 7: superficial femoral in the adductor canal; 8: superficial femoral about to pierce the adductor hiatus.

branches until it enters the popliteal fossa where it gives off an important late branch, the descending genicular, which contributes to the collateral circulation at the level of the knee (Figure 6-10).

In its proximal course, the CFA gives off the profunda femoris artery (PFA) from its lateral side about 4 cm below the inguinal ligament. **The circumflex branches from the proximal part of the PFA** and forms the collateral network of the upper leg and hip along with the branches from the IIA (Figure 6-9). Similarly, perforating branches arising from the distal part of the PFA form the collateral network of the knee and lower leg with the branches of the popliteal and tibial vessels.

At the distal, posterior aspect of the femur, the SFA passes through the adductor hiatus to become the popliteal artery (Figure 6-10). The

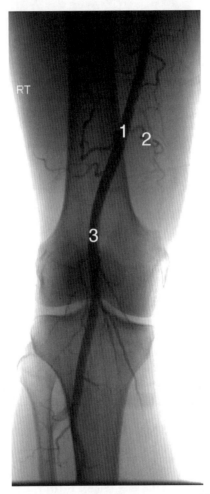

Figure **6-10** **Right femoro-popliteal system.** 1: superficial femoral piercing the adductor hiatus; 2: descending genicular branch; 3: popliteal.

popliteal artery then trifurcates into the anterior tibial artery (AT), peroneal artery, and posterior tibial artery (PT) (Figure 6-11). The AT leaves the main popliteal body by piercing through the interosseous membrane anteriorly. The popliteal then continues as a short posterior segment called the tibioperoneal (TP) trunk. As it exits out of the

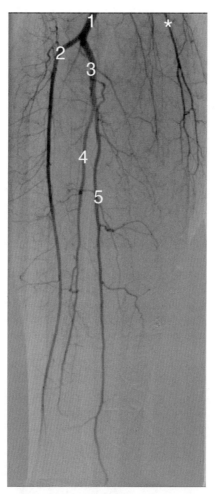

Figure **6-11** **Right popliteal and infrapopliteal system.** 1: popliteal; 2: anterior tibial; 3: tibioperoneal trunk; 4: peroneal artery; 5: posterior tibial artery. *Also seen is the descending genicular branch arising proximally from the distal superficial femoral artery.

popliteal fossa, the TP trunk gives rise to the peroneal artery laterally, which runs between the interosseous membrane and the fibula and terminates above the level of the ankle joint. The TP trunk then continues on medially as the PT.

The arterial supply of the foot is via continuations of the AT and PT (Figure 6-12). The AT becomes the dorsalis pedis artery as it crosses midway between the malleoli and lies over the planar surface of the foot. The PT courses posterior to the medial malleolus and terminates on the

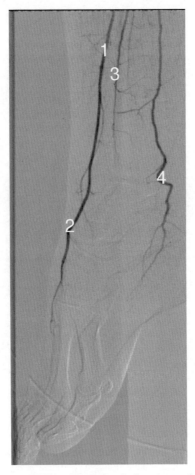

Figure **6-12**   **Right ankle and foot circulation.** 1: anterior tibial; 2: dorsalis pedis; 3: peroneal; 4: posterior tibial.

plantar surface of the foot as medial and lateral plantar branches. These foot arteries form important collaterals among themselves when their proximal parent vessels are occluded.

Angiography: Prior to angiography some general rules should be followed: (1) access is typically obtained in the CFA contralateral to the limb with worse symptoms or noninvasively tested parameters; (2) a low-osmolar, nonionic contrast is ideal to minimize contrast-related limb discomfort; (3) sequential static overlapping DSA at multiple levels provides the most comprehensive angiographic evaluation of each limb. A significant limitation of peripheral angiography is the quantity of contrast used and excessive radiation exposure.

Angiography of the aortic bifurcation and iliac arteries may be performed with power contrast injection using a 4-Fr. to 5-Fr. pigtail catheter, Omni Flush catheter, or Straight Flush catheter. Typically, a power

Troubleshooting

1. Artery is cannulated with good blood return but guidewire cannot be advanced beyond a certain point: Given the possibility of severe peripheral arterial disease (PAD) including total occlusions, the needle should be exchanged for a small (4-Fr.) micropuncture sheath and then contrast should gently be injected to assess for occlusion, tortuosity, or dissection. Never advance a wire that does not have a freely mobile tip.

2. Image quality is compromised by motion artifact: Consider taping the patient's feet to maintain stability. The patient should always be instructed not to move or breathe during DSA acquisition.

3. Too much scatter or brightness compromising image quality: In contrast to coronary angiography, angiographic images of the periphery are extremely sensitive to ambient light. Thus, placement of a central wedge filter between the legs and two lateral wedge filters placed lateral to each leg can greatly enhance image quality by ensuring focused penetration of the x-rays in the area of interest.

4. Poor opacification of infrapopliteal vasculature: This can occur if the site of injection is too proximal (e.g., EIA). Positioning the diagnostic catheter into the ipsilateral distal SFA or sometimes even in the ipsilateral popliteal artery can prevent this problem.

5. Overlap of arterial bed in the foot: The dorsal and plantar arterial arches can have significant overlap making the identification of lesions difficult. This issue can be overcome in most cases by external rotation and dorsiflexion of the foot which separates the dorsal and plantar arterial supply.

injection of 15 mL per second for a total of 30 mL is sufficient to adequately visualize the aortic bifurcation and pelvic arteries. Angiographic views are taken in the standard PA projection; but in the case of tortuous vessels or eccentric lesions, angulated views (RAO or LAO) may be needed (Figure 6-8). For the CIA, an oblique view is obtained with 30° to 45° contralateral angulation. Alternatively for the EIA, ipsilateral oblique angulation between 30° and 45° is preferred.

Angiography of the lower extremity and its distal runoff is best done via a selective approach. As mentioned above, access is obtained contralateral to the limb of interest. In one technique, a side-hole flush catheter such as an Omni Flush, Universal Flush, or Grollman catheter is advanced into the abdominal aorta through the access sheath over a soft 0.035 wire such as a Wholey or Tiger wire. The flush catheter is then retracted slowly until the catheter tip gently hooks the contralateral CIA while the body of the catheter hugs the aortic bifurcation. The flush catheter is then advanced over the wire to the contralateral EIA or CFA where it is used for selective injection. One limitation of this technique is that the flush catheter may not be able to be easily advanced through tortuous or calcified anatomy. Another common technique involves using an IMA catheter to hook the contralateral CIA by retracting it slowly over the 0.035 wire and withdrawing the wire into the catheter at the level of the iliac bifurcation. The wire can then be advanced down the contralateral iliac distally; and the catheter can be exchanged for a straight flush or multipurpose catheter which can then be advanced over the wire to the level of the CFA for selective injection and run-off angiography. If the ipsilateral lower extremity needs to be imaged, contrast injection directly through the arterial sheath in the CFA usually allows for adequate visualization of the distal vasculature.

Lower extremity arterial segments are then imaged sequentially using the following general scheme: (1) origin of CFA to distal SFA (above knee); (2) distal SFA to distal to posterior tibial and peroneal bifurcation (knee); (3) distal popliteal to distal AT/PT (below knee); and (4) distal AT/PT to terminal branches forming the plantar arterial arch (foot). Ipsilateral PA views are standard for SFA and popliteal arteries; however, the AT, TP trunk, and PT should be examined in an ipsilateral 15° to 30° view. The foot should be examined in the contralateral oblique view at 15° to 20°. The CFA bifurcation, including the ostia of the SFA and PFA, can be optimally viewed at an ipsilateral oblique angulation of 20° to 30° (Figure 6-9). **Similarly, a true lateral allows better assessment of the distal popliteal, whereas an ipsilateral oblique angulation of about 30° optimizes visualization of the infrapopliteal trifurcation** (Figures 6-10 and 6-11). Typically, a "long column of contrast" (e.g., rate of 3 mL per second for 5–10 mL injection) is required for below-the-knee vessels. As the imaging plane is moved down the lower extremity, a slight delay (2–4 sec) between injection and DSA activation is recommended to account for transit time and minimize radiation exposure.

Complications

1. Access related: Complications related to access such as hematoma, pseudoaneurysm, arteriovenous fistula, dissection, or retroperitoneal bleed remain the most common form of complications with all angiographic procedures. **The incidence of vascular complications is up to 1% in coronary series but is higher in patients with peripheral vascular disease.** Vascular complications during peripheral angiography are evaluated and managed in the same way as vascular complications occurring with coronary angiography. These are discussed in detail in Chapters 8 and 9.

2. Angiography related: Complications resulting from wire and catheter manipulation are rare with diagnostic angiography; but when they do occur, they require prompt recognition and management with pharmacologic and mechanical therapies. These include vessel dissection, perforation, or vessel closure due to plaque shift. Some of the clinical syndromes arising from these complications are discussed below.

   • Acute limb ischemia: This can result from thrombus formation on equipment especially in long cases or when meticulous discard and flushing is not performed. Percutaneous mechanical thrombectomy should be promptly attempted by a qualified interventionalist and can be supplemented with adjunctive thrombolytic or glycoprotein IIb/IIIa therapy.

   • Cerebreovascular accident: These usually manifest within a few hours after the procedure and can be in the form of a transient ischemic attack or a stroke. If the patient has signs and/or symptoms of a neurologic event during or following the procedure, do not move the patient from the catheterization table. Cerebral angiography should be performed immediately with comparison to the initial baseline angiograms. This scenario highlights the importance of baseline cerebral angiographic imaging. If the repeat cerebral angiogram is normal, then the prognosis is usually excellent. However, if a large artery (2–2.5 mm) occlusion occurs due to distal embolization, recanalization should be attempted by a qualified interventionalist using directed thrombolytics or mechanical extraction.

   • Intracranial hemorrhage (ICH): This feared complication is exceedingly rare with just diagnostic angiography. However, if ICH does occur, it demands emergent assessment by a neurovascular surgeon.

3. Miscellaneous: Other general complications such as a radiation injury, acute renal insufficiency, and sedation-related complications are evaluated and managed as with coronary angiography.

Suggested Reading

Criqui MH. Peripheral arterial disease and subsequent cardiovascular mortality: a strong and consistent association. *Circulation.* 1990;82:2246–2247.

Bhatt DL, Steg PG, Ohman EM, et al; REACH Registry Investigators. International prevalence, recognition, and treatment of cardiovascular risk factors in outpatients with atherothrombosis. *JAMA.* 2006;295:180–189.

Hirsch AT, Criqui MH, Treat-Jacobson D, et al. Peripheral arterial disease detection, awareness, and treatment in primary care. *JAMA.* 2001;286:1317–1324.

Norgren L, Hiatt WR, Dormandy JA, et al. Inter-society consensus for the management of peripheral arterial disease (TASC II). *Eur J Vasc Endovasc Surg.* 2007;33(suppl 1):S1–S75.

Hirsch AT, Haskal ZJ, Hertzer NR, et al. ACC/AHA 2005 guidelines for the management of patients with peripheral arterial disease (lower extremity, renal, mesenteric, and abdominal aortic): executive summary a collaborative report from the American Association for Vascular Surgery/Society for Vascular Surgery, Society for Cardiovascular Angiography and Interventions, Society for Vascular Medicine and Biology, Society of Interventional Radiology, and the ACC/AHA Task Force on Practice Guidelines (Writing Committee to Develop Guidelines for the Management of Patients With Peripheral Arterial Disease) endorsed by the American Association of Cardiovascular and Pulmonary Rehabilitation; National Heart, Lung, and Blood Institute; Society for Vascular Nursing; TransAtlantic Inter-Society Consensus; and Vascular Disease Foundation. *J Am Coll Cardiol.* 2006; 47:1239–1312.

Uflacker R, ed. *Atlas of Vascular Anatomy: An Angiographic Approach.* 2nd ed. Philadelphia: Lippincott Williams & Wilkins; 2006.

Valji K, ed. *Vascular and Interventional Radiology.* 2nd ed. Philadelphia: Saunders Elsevier; 2006.

Cassserly IP, Sachar R, Yadav JS, eds. *Manual of Peripheral Vascular Intervention.* 1st ed. Philadelphia: Lippincott Williams & Wilkins; 2005.

Khoury M, Batra S, Berg R, et al. Influence of arterial access sites and interventional procedures on vascular complications after cardiac catheterizations. *Am J Surg.* 1992;164:205–209.

CHAPTER 7

Hemodynamics in the Cath Lab

Brian W. Hardaway, Wilson H. Tang, and Frederick A. Heupler, Jr.

Hemodynamic data are an important part of every diagnostic catheterization, particularly in patients with cardiomyopathies, valvular disorders, and pericardial disease. The measurement of hemodynamics utilizes pressure, oximetry, and temperature differences to derive functional information about the heart. To fully understand hemodynamics, one must first learn how to make proper measurements, calculate derived values, and interpret the results in relation to specific disease conditions.

Methodologies of Hemodynamic Measurements

Pressure Measurements: The most accurate method for measuring pressure in the heart is to utilize a system with the pressure transducer (usually a strain gauge type) located at the exact location of interest. However, while catheters with a pressure transducer at the tip are available, they are too expensive to be used routinely and are generally only used for research purposes. Thus, the most common method of measuring pressure in the cardiac catheterization lab utilizes a system incorporating a fluid-filled catheter connected through a manifold to a pressure transducer. This system, however, has several characteristics that influence its fidelity and its accuracy. Because the pressure waveform is transmitted through fluid until it reaches the transducer outside the body, there is both a time delay and a dampening of the pressure signal that usually filters out the high frequency components. Underdamping of the system can be a problem especially if air bubbles are present in the system (Figure 7-1). Other common sources of error are listed in Table 7-1.

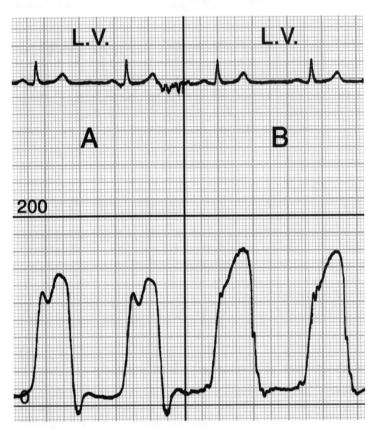

Figure **7-1** **A)** Normal pressure waveform. **B)** Pressure underdamping caused by an air bubble in the tubing. This produces high frequency oscillations that result in the peak pressures appearing higher.

Oximetry Measurements: Oximetry measurements are most commonly performed to measure cardiac output utilizing the Fick method (described later in this chapter) and to rule out a left-to-right shunt (described later in this chapter). Oximetry measures the oxygen saturation of blood. The oxygen content of blood can then be calculated.

Oxygen content ~Hgb(g/dL) × 1.36(mLO$_2$/g Hgb) × Sat

where Hgb is hemoglobin in grams per deciliter; 1.36 is the oxygen carrying capacity of blood in milliliters of oxygen per gram of hemoglobin; and Sat is the oxygen saturation of the blood. The dissolved

Table **7-1**	Common Sources of Error in Hemodynamic Measurements	
Source of Error	**Correct Technique**	**Common Example of Error**
Transducer position	At level of mid-right atrium, halfway up the body between spine and sternum	↓ Pressure recorded if positioned too high
Catheter bore	Maximize catheter bore size	
Catheter length	Minimize length of tubing	
Kink in tubing	Replace tubing or catheter	
Fluid viscosity	Catheter should be filled with normal saline, avoid contrast	Contrast in tubing
Air in system	Flush catheters and manifold to avoid presence of air bubbles	Air bubble at connection points or at transducer
Tip positioning	Reposition catheter	"Catheter whip"
Stable arrhythmias	Average measurements over several beats to obtain an average	

Troubleshooting

Inserting PA Catheter

1. Obtain vascular accesses, typically with an 8-Fr. sheath, allowing passage of the 7-Fr. PA (Swan-Ganz) catheter. Typically, if the pulmonary artery (PA) catheter is guided solely by pressure tracings to advance it to wedge position, the right internal jugular vein and the left subclavian vein provide the most direct anatomic routes to the pulmonary artery that matches the natural curve of the catheter.

2. Inflate the balloon at the tip of the catheter under water to ensure no air leak.

3. Make sure that all lumens of the PA catheter are flushed.

4. Zero the pressure transducer at the level of the mid-right atrium.

5. Connect the PA catheter's distal port to the pressure transducer. Make sure that there are no bubbles in the tubing or the catheter.

6. Advance the catheter 20 cm through the sheath prior to balloon inflation to ensure the catheter tip clears the sheath. Do not advance if any resistance is met.

7. Beware of arrhythmias especially after the catheter crosses the tricuspid valve, primarily premature ventricular contractions (PVCs), and non-sustained ventricular tachycardia (NSVT). In the setting of underlying LBBB, the catheter may induce complete heart block. In the setting of myocardial infarction, the catheter may induce ventricular fibrillation.

8. Monitor pressures as the catheter is being advanced through the right atrium (RA), right ventricle (RV), and PA to wedge position. Be careful not to overwedge.

9. Do not pull back the catheter with the balloon inflated. Damage to valves, either pulmonary or tricuspid may result.

oxygen in blood is generally negligible in these calculations and is usually ignored.

Temperature Measurements: A thermistor is mounted at the tip of the pulmonary artery catheter to measure the temperature of the fluid as it passes through the pulmonary artery. Temperature is most commonly used to calculate cardiac output using the thermodilution technique, which is a variant of indicator dilution. Cold saline is injected through an opening in the catheter 25 to 30 cm proximal to the tip. The temperature is measured as a function of time, and temperature change can be used to calculate cardiac output (see "Cardiac Output" section).

Hemodynamic Measurements in Clinical Scenarios: See Figures 7-2 through 7-6.

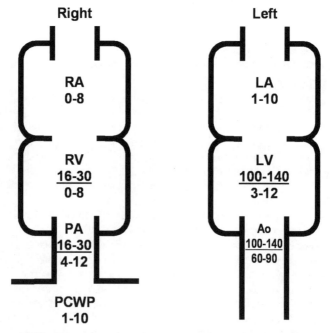

Figure **7-2**   Normal hemodynamic pressure measurements in various cardiac chambers. RA, mean right atrial pressure; RV, right ventricular pressure; PA, pulmonary artery pressure; PCW, pulmonary capillary wedge pressure; LA, mean left atrial pressure; LV, left ventricular pressure.

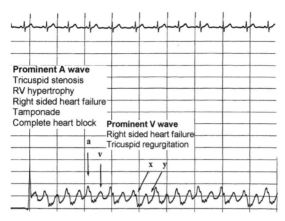

Figure **7-3** **Normal RA pressures.** Right atrial pressure is the same as central venous pressure and is equal to right ventricular diastolic pressure. "a" wave, right atrial systole; "x" descent, right atrial relaxation; "v" wave, right atrial filling during ventricular systole; "y"-descent, right atrial emptying. Usually, the "a" wave is higher than the "v" wave in normal patients. Giant "a" waves are seen in right-sided heart failure with a stiff right ventricle. Cannon "a" waves are seen in complete heart block when the right atrium contracts against a closed tricuspid valve. (Note: The distance between horizontal lines is 4 mm Hg, and the time between vertical lines is 1 second.) (From Topol EJ, Califf RM, et al. Textbook of Cardiovascular Medicine, 3rd Edition. Philadelphia: Lippincott Williams & Wilkins, 2006.)

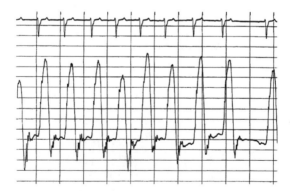

Figure **7-4** **Normal RV pressures.** Right ventricular systolic pressures are elevated with right-sided heart failure, pulmonary valve stenosis, and pulmonary hypertension. Right ventricular diastolic pressures are elevated with cardiac tamponade and increased right ventricular stiffness. (Note that the distance between horizontal lines is 4 mm Hg and the time between vertical lines is 1 second.) (From Topol EJ, Califf RM, et al. Textbook of Cardiovascular Medicine, 3rd Edition. Philadelphia: Lippincott Williams & Wilkins, 2006.)

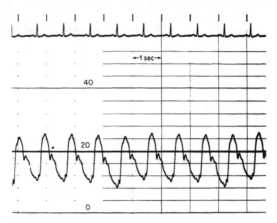

Figure **7-5**　**PA pressures.** Pulmonary artery pressures are elevated with left-sided heart failure, lung disease, and pulmonary vascular disease. In pulmonary vascular disease, the pulmonary artery diastolic pressure can be significantly higher than the pulmonary capillary wedge pressure. This finding is most commonly found in primary pulmonary hypertension, chronic pulmonary embolism, and Eisenmenger syndrome with intracardiac shunts. (Note: The distance between horizontal lines is 4 mm Hg, and the time between vertical lines is 1 second.) (From Willard JE, Lange RA, Hillis LD. Cardiac catheterization. In: Kloner RA, ed. The guide to cardiology, 3rd. Ed. New York: Le Jacq Communications, 1995:145–164.)

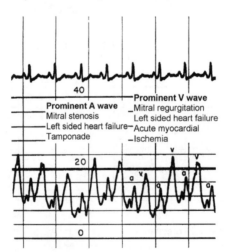

Figure **7-6**　Pulmonary capillary wedge pressures. "a" wave, left atrial systole; "v" wave, left atrial filling during ventricular systole. (Note: The distance between horizontal lines is 4 mm Hg, and the time between vertical lines is 1 second.) (Adapted from Willard JE, Lange RA, Hillis LD. Cardiac catheterization. In: Kloner RA, ed. The guide to cardiology, 3rd. Ed. New York: Le Jacq Communications, 1995:145–164.)

PRESSURE GRADIENTS ACROSS STENOSES: Measuring pressure gradients across stenotic valves is an important process in determining the need for surgical intervention particularly when the hemodynamics as measured by noninvasive means are in question. The valve orifice area can often be estimated by a formula that was developed by Dr. Richard Gorlin if the mean pressure gradient, cardiac output, and the systolic ejection time are known; particularly if the patient is not in a low cardiac output state:

$$\text{Valve orifice area (VOA) in cm}^2 = \frac{\text{cardiac output(L/min)}}{44.3 \times (K) \times \text{heart rate} \times (\text{SEP or DFP}) \times \sqrt{\Delta P(\text{mm Hg})}}$$

where SEP is the systolic ejection period in aortic stenosis (length of time blood is ejected from LV every beat); DFP is the diastolic filling period in mitral stenosis (length of time blood filling LV every beat); ΔP is the mean pressure gradient; constant $(K = 0.85)$ is added in mitral stenosis.

The Hakki formula is a simplified derivation of the Gorlin equation:

$$\text{Valve orifice area (VOA) in cm}^2 = \sqrt{\frac{\text{cardiac output(L/min)}}{\text{pressure gradient(mm Hg)}}}$$

The Angel correction mandates that the above result be divided by 1.35 for a heart rate <75 beats per minute in the setting of mitral stenosis, or >90 beats per minute in the setting of aortic stenosis.

Caution is advised when using the Hakki formula if coexisting aortic regurgitation or mitral regurgitation is present as this will cause underestimation of the aortic valve area and mitral valve area respectively.

Aortic Stenosis: **The normal orifice area of the aortic valve is 3 to 4 cm².** The aortic valve can become significantly narrowed prior to the onset of symptoms or even hemodynamic significance.

Aortic Valve Orifice Areas

Normal aortic orifice area	3–4 cm²
Mild stenosis	>1.5 cm²
Moderate stenosis	1.0–1.5 cm²
Severe stenosis	<1.0 cm²

The most accurate method for measuring aortic valve gradients is by obtaining simultaneous pressure measurements from the left

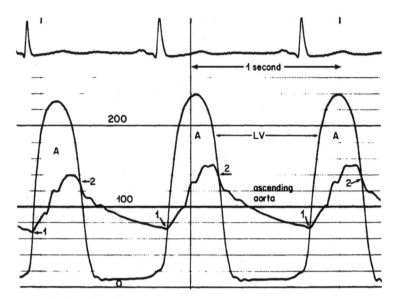

Figure **7-7**   Simultaneous pressure tracings of left ventricle and ascending aorta, demonstrating the significant gradient across the aortic valve. (From Willard JE, Lange RA, Hillis LD. Cardiac catheterization. In: Kloner RA, ed. The guide to cardiology, 3rd. Ed. New York: Le Jacq Communications, 1995:145–164.)

ventricle and the ascending aorta (Figure 7-7**).** This method allows the calculation of the mean gradient by direct measurement from both recordings. The easiest way to accomplish this is to use a dual-lumen pigtail catheter, which permits simultaneous measurement of pressures in the LV and ascending aorta.

Alternatively, a long arterial sheath can be placed in the descending thoracic aorta, and pressure measured from the sideport. The femoral artery pressure is also often substituted for this measurement. The peak femoral artery pressure is usually higher than the peak aortic root pressure due to reflected pressure waves seen in the periphery, thus using the femoral artery results in underestimation of the pressure gradient. This can be somewhat compensated by measuring the pressure difference between the catheter at the ascending aorta and the sidearm of the femoral artery sheath, and subtracting the difference.

A more commonly utilized method involves pullback of the catheter from the left ventricle into the ascending aorta. This technique yields a "peak-to-peak" gradient between the maximum aortic pressure and the

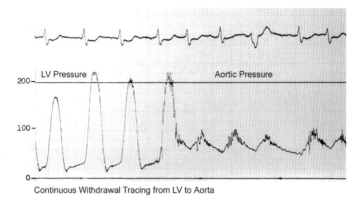

Continuous Withdrawal Tracing from LV to Aorta

Figure **7-8**   Pressure tracing of the pullback across the aortic valve.

maximum left ventricular pressure (Figure 7-8). Each of these peaks occurs at different points in time, however, and this measurement is only
an estimate of the mean gradient. In addition, in patients with severe
aortic stenosis, the catheter itself may take up a significant fraction of
the orifice area, resulting in worsened stenosis and increased gradients.

The Gorlin and Hakki formulas can be used to estimate the valve orifice area, but may be inaccurate in severe aortic stenosis with low-output
states. The accuracy of the formula is flow-dependent and will result in
small orifice areas, despite low gradients, if the flow across the aortic
valve is low. This is frequently observed in patients with severe systolic
LV dysfunction.

If maneuvers to increase cardiac output (i.e., exercise, dobutamine,
nitroprusside) are performed on this subset of patients and a significant
increase in the estimated valve orifice area is observed (usually resulting
in a valve area >1 cm^2) this is termed "pseudostenosis." Failure of the
estimated valve orifice area to significantly increase with these measures
implies either true severe aortic stenosis (increase in aortic valve pressure
gradients with maneuvers) or poor left ventricular contractile reserve (no
significant increase in aortic valve pressures with maneuvers).

Mitral Stenosis: **The normal mitral valve orifice area is 4 to 6 cm^2.**
Significant narrowing can occur prior to hemodynamic compromise.
When the valve area falls to $\sim$2.0 cm^2, the left atrial pressures will start increasing to maintain cardiac output. Valve areas less than 1.0 cm^2 frequently require some intervention.

Troubleshooting

Calculating Valve Area in Aortic Stenosis

68-year-old male:

CO = 4800 mL/min
HR = 80 beats per minute
SEP = 0.35
Mean AV gradient = 80 mm Hg

Gorlin formula:

$$\text{Valve orifice area (VOA)} = \frac{CO/(HR)(SEP)}{44.3\ (k)\ \sqrt{\Delta P}}$$

$$VOA = \frac{4800/(80)(0.35)}{44.3(\sqrt{80})} = 0.4\ cm^2$$

Hakki formula:

$$VOA = \frac{CO(L/min)}{\sqrt{\Delta P}}$$

$$VOA = \frac{4.8}{(\sqrt{80})} = 0.5\ cm^2$$

Mitral Valve Orifice Areas

Normal mitral orifice area	4–6 cm^2
Mild stenosis	>1.6 cm^2
Moderate stenosis	1.1–1.5 cm^2
Severe stenosis	<1.0 cm^2

The "Gold Standard" for determination of mitral valve gradients remains simultaneous direct LA pressure (via interatrial septostomy) and LV pressure measurements. Frequently, however, direct LA pressure measurement is substituted by PCWP measurement (Figure 7-9). Caution is advised when interpreting simultaneous PCWP/LV pressure tracings for the determination of the mitral valve gradient as there is a temporal delay between early left atrial emptying and the corresponding y-descent seen on PCWP tracings which leads to overestimation of the mean mitral gradient. Some heart catheterization laboratories have computerized algorithms to compensate for this overestimation.

The Gorlin equation is also used in this instance, except that the diastolic filling period (Figure 7-10) is substituted in lieu of the systolic ejection

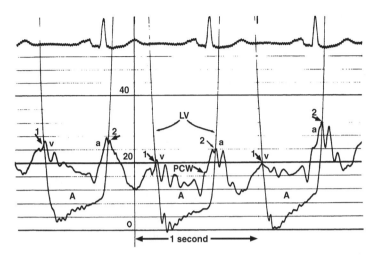

Figure **7-9** Simultaneous pressure tracings of PCWP and the LV demonstrating the gradient across the mitral valve and the slow y-descent of the PCW pressure tracing. (From Willard JE, Lange RA, Hillis LD. Cardiac catheterization. In: Kloner RA, ed. The guide to cardiology, 3rd ed. New York: Le Jacq Communications, 1995: 145–164.)

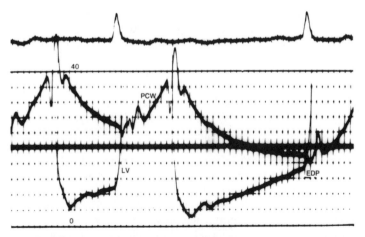

Figure **7-10** Diastolic filling period used to calculate the mitral valve area.

Troubleshooting

Calculating Valve Area in Mitral Stenosis

37-year-old male:

    CO = 5000 mL/min
    HR = 76 beats per minute
    DFP = 0.4
    Mean MV gradient = 20 mm Hg

Gorlin:

$$\text{Valve orifice area (VOA)} = \frac{CO/(HR)(DFP)}{44.3\ (k)\sqrt{\Delta P}}$$

where k = 0.85 (for the mitral valve)

$$VOA = \frac{5000/(76)(0.4)}{44.3(0.85)(\sqrt{20})} = 1.0\ cm^2$$

Hakki:

$$VOA = \frac{CO(L/min)}{\sqrt{\Delta P}}$$

$$VOA = \frac{5.0}{(\sqrt{20})} = 1.1\ cm^2$$

period used in AS, and that an empiric constant of 0.85 is added to the equation. Concomitant mitral regurgitation with mitral stenosis will affect this calculation, and usually will underestimate the true orifice area.

Hypertrophic Obstructive Cardiomyopathy (HOCM): In HOCM, the obstruction lies below the aortic valve and may be dynamic, with little or no resting gradient. The pullback to measure the peak-to-peak pressure should start at the ventricular apex and proceed through the left ventricular outflow tract and through the valve. In typical HOCM, there will be a gradient from the ventricular apex to the LVOT, but no gradient across the valve (Figure 7-11). In Yamaguchi's variant (apical LVH), no gradient will be noted, although the classic spade-like appearance may be observed with left ventriculography.

If a significant resting gradient is not appreciated, then provocative maneuvers can be performed to unmask an intraventricular gradient. The most common maneuvers include Valsalva, nitroglycerin administration, amyl nitrite inhalation, or PVC induction. In patients suspected of HOCM, the immediate post-PVC beat is characterized by an increase in

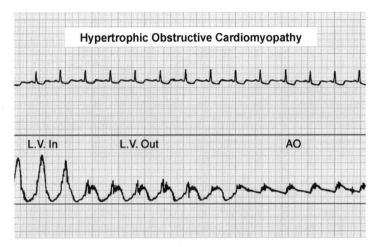

Figure **7-11**   Pullback from LV apex to LV outflow tract demonstrating an intraventricular gradient consistent with HOCM.

contractility which leads to an increase in the dynamic LVOT obstruction resulting in a decrease in stroke volume and hence a decrease in pulse pressure as compared to the beat immediately preceding the PVC. This is known as the Brockenbrough–Braunwald–Morrow sign (Figure 7-12). Alternatively, in the case of a fixed obstruction (i.e., Aortic Stenosis) the post-PVC beat is characterized by an increase in contractility resulting in an increase in stroke volume and hence an increase in pulse pressure as compared to the pre-PVC beat.

Intracardiac Pressure Waveforms

Mitral and Tricuspid Regurgitation: The hemodynamic hallmarks of mitral regurgitation are increased left atrial pressure and reduced cardiac output. A prominent *v* wave is suggestive of, but not specific to, mitral regurgitation (Figure 7-13).

Cardiac Tamponade: A pericardial effusion that results in hemodynamic compromise causes tamponade. With regard to hemodynamic measurements, there is eventual diastolic equalization of pressures in all cardiac chambers (CVP = RVEDP = PCWP = LVEDP), usually associated with pulsus paradoxus (exaggerated inspiratory fall in arterial pressures of greater than 10 mm Hg), a fall in cardiac output, and hypotension. Pulsus paradoxus, however, is neither sensitive nor specific for

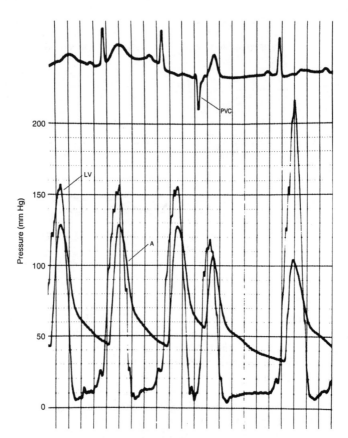

Figure **7-12** **Brockenbrough–Braunwald–Morrow sign.** The gradient across the aortic valve is increased in the postextrasystolic beat, with a reduction in aortic or systemic pressure. This accentuation of the gradient is either small or absent in a fixed obstruction/valvular aortic stenosis.

tamponade, and may be found in constrictive pericarditis, pulmonary embolism, and COPD. On the pressure tracings, there may be a prominent x-descent with a blunted y-descent in addition to the diastolic equalization of pressures (Figure 7-14).

Constrictive versus Restrictive Physiology: The diagnosis of constrictive pericarditis may be difficult. Differentiating constrictive pericarditis from restrictive cardiomyopathy is even harder. From a hemodynamic standpoint constrictive pericarditis is characterized by equalization of

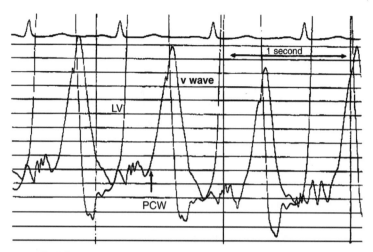

Figure **7-13**   **Severe mitral regurgitation.** The V wave in the PCW tracing is very prominent in this case, and the y-descent is sharp. (From Topol EJ, ed. *Textbook of Cardiovascular Medicine.* Philadelphia, PA: Lippincott Williams & Wilkins; 2002.)

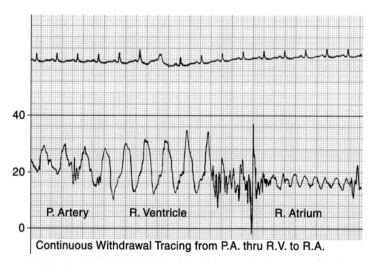

Figure **7-14   Cardiac tamponade, with a large pericardial effusion.** Note the diastolic equalization of pressures in the RV and RA positions.

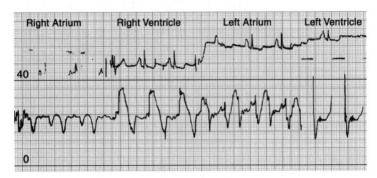

Figure **7-15** **Constrictive pericarditis.** A classic "W" or "M" pattern is seen in the right atrial tracing.

diastolic pressures and ventricular interdependence. The classic hemodynamic criteria for constrictive pericarditis are (1) less than 5 mm Hg difference between the LVEDP and RVEDP, (2) PA pressure less than 60 mm Hg, and (3) RVEDP/RVSP ratio greater than 30%. Other findings observed on pressure tracings of constrictive pericarditis include a "dip and plateau" pattern in the ventricular pressure tracings, an "M or W" pattern in the atrial tracing, and an elevation of the mean right atrial pressure during inspiration, none of these features is either sensitive or specific for the diagnosis of constriction (Figure 7-15).

During inspiration there is an increase in right-sided flow and pressure. The constraining effect of the pericardium on right ventricular expansion in diastole causes interventricular septal bowing toward the left ventricle. This septal bowing effectively leads to a decrease in left ventricular preload and subsequently cardiac output. The reverse happens with expiration where LV flow and pressure increases and interventricular septal bowing toward the right ventricle occurs causing a decrease in right-sided pressures. This concept of ventricular interdependence in constrictive pericarditis can be demonstrated by obtaining simultaneous RV and LV pressure tracings. Discordance of the LV and RV systolic pressures will be observed during the respiratory cycle (Figure 7-16). **Respiratory discordance between the LV and RV systolic pressure is more sensitive than classic hemodynamic criteria for differentiating constrictive pericarditis from restrictive myocardial disease in the majority of patients, but it still remains less than 80% sensitive. More recently, the respiratory changes in the areas under the curves of the RV and LV pressure tracings have been shown to be more reliable than the systolic pressure changes. The "Systolic Area Index" is the ratio of the RV area (mm Hg × seconds) to the LV**

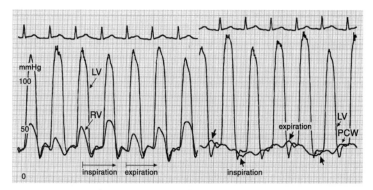

Figure **7-16   Constrictive pericarditis.** Ventricular interdependence and respiratory variation are seen in this example.

area (mm Hg × seconds) in inspiration versus expiration. A systolic area index greater than 1.1 has a sensitivity and positive predictive value greater than 95% for differentiating constrictive pericarditis from restrictive myocardial disease.

Shunt Calculation: Shunts can be localized and quantified using oximetry, indocyanine green dye, and angiography. The most common method used clinically is oximetry. In the location of the shunt, blood usually flows from the left-sided (higher pressure) chamber to the right-sided (lower pressure) chamber (left-to-right shunt), with abnormally high oxygen saturation in that chamber and all chambers distal. The level where this "step-up" in oxygen saturation is detected identifies where the shunt exists. **A "step-up" is considered significant if it is >7% from the vena cava to the right atrium and >5% from the right atrium to the right ventricle or >5% from the right ventricle to the pulmonary artery.**

The quantification of shunting is determined by calculating the shunt fraction, which in left-to-right shunts is the Qp/Qs (the ratio of pulmonary to systemic blood flow). Oxygen saturations should be drawn in the superior vena cava, inferior vena cava, right atrium (three sites), right ventricle (three sites), pulmonary artery, and aorta.

$$\frac{Qp}{Qs} = \frac{O_2 \, \text{sat(systemic arterial)} - O_2 \, \text{sat(systemic mixed venous)}}{O_2 \, \text{sat(pulmonary venous)} - O_2 \, \text{sat(pulmonary arterial)}}$$

Adding 3 × SVC saturation to the IVC saturation, and dividing the sum by 4 calculates the mixed venous saturation.

Troubleshooting

Shunt Calculation

61-year-old male with an ASD and the following O_2 saturations:

Femoral artery = 98% (systemic arterial and pulmonary venous)
SVC = 69%
IVC = 73%
PA = 80%

$$MVO_2 = \frac{(3)(0.69) + (0.73)}{4} = 0.70 \,(\text{systemic mixed venous})$$

$$\frac{Qp}{Qs} = \frac{O_2 \, Sat(\text{systemic arterial}) - O_2 \, Sat(\text{systemic mixed venous})}{O_2 \, Sat(\text{pulmonary venous}) - O_2 \, Sat(\text{pulmonary arterial})}$$

$$\frac{Qp}{Qs} = \frac{0.98 - 0.70}{0.98 - 0.80} = 1.55$$

Remember:
Qp/Qs: <1.5 = small
1.5–2.0 = medium
>2.0 = large

Minimal Qp/Qs Reliably Detected

1.5–1.9 at level of atrium
1.3–1.5 at level of ventricle
1.3 at level of great vessels

Shunts are small if the Qp/Qs <1.5, moderate if the Qp/Qs is between 1.5 and 2.0, and large if the Qp/Qs is >2.

Right-to-Left Shunts: Right-to-left shunts cannot be localized or quantified using a standard right heart catheterization. Sampling must be done at the pulmonary vein level as well as the chamber of interest (e.g., left atrium) to determine if a "step-down" in saturation is found. This technique usually necessitates a trans-septal puncture.

Cardiac Performance

Cardiac Output: The primary purpose of the heart is to deliver oxygenated blood to the peripheral tissues. Cardiac output is measured clinically in two ways, the thermodilution and the Fick methods. Cardiac output can also be indirectly estimated with left ventriculography. Cardiac output is affected by several different factors including age, body size, and metabolic demands. To normalize resting cardiac output among different body sizes, the cardiac index is used:

$$\text{Cardiac index}(\text{L/min/m}^2) = \frac{\text{CO}(\text{L/min})}{\text{BSA}(\text{m}^2)}$$

where

$$\text{BSA (body surface area)} = \frac{\sqrt{[\text{height(cm)} \times \text{weight(kg)}]}}{3600}$$

Thermodilution Method: **The thermodilution technique is based on indicator dilution methods**. This method utilizes a bolus injection of a known amount of a substance, and followed by measurement of the concentration of this substance downstream as a function of time. The concentration–time curve can then be used to determine the cardiac output. While this technique has been used with several different indicators, for example, indocyanine green, **the most common indicator used today is room temperature saline**, with the temperature difference between saline and blood measured in lieu of concentration. The temperature is measured with a thermistor usually at the level of the injectate bag and at the tip of the catheter. While this usually provides a reasonably accurate result, if the temperature of the saline is increased between the injectate bag and the injection port, the measurement can be falsely elevated. Most commonly this occurs because the saline is heated by the operator's hand while in the injection syringe. In low-output states, the saline gets warmed by the blood and heart prior to reaching the thermistor, which may result in inaccurate calculations. Valvular abnormalities, such as tricuspid or pulmonic regurgitation, or intracardiac shunting will also affect the thermodilution cardiac output.

Fick Method: Adolph Fick, in 1870, developed a principle that demonstrated that **the total uptake or release of any substance by an organ is the product of blood flow to the organ and the arteriovenous**

Troubleshooting

Common Pitfalls in Measuring Cardiac Output
1. Warming the saline in the syringe with your hand prior to injection in the thermodilution method.
2. Not measuring cardiac outputs at the same time that pressure measurements are done.

concentration difference of the substance. In common clinical practice, the organ to which this is applied is the lungs, and the substance is oxygen. This method calculates pulmonary blood flow, which in the absence of intracardiac shunts, equals systemic blood flow. Thus, systemic blood flow equals oxygen consumption divided by the pulmonary arteriovenous oxygen difference. The arteriovenous oxygen difference is calculated by subtracting the oxygen content of mixed venous blood, usually pulmonary arterial blood in most clinical settings, from pulmonary venous blood, which is estimated by systemic arterial blood. The oxygen content equals oxygen saturation (%) multiplied by 1.36 mL O_2/g hemoglobin (oxygen carrying capacity of hemoglobin) multiplied by hemoglobin (g/100 mL blood). The term for dissolved oxygen in the blood is usually negligible and therefore dropped.

$$\text{Fick CO(L/min)} =$$

$$\frac{\text{oxygen consumption(mL/min)}}{(\text{arterial} - \text{venous } O_2 \text{ sat}) \times 1.36 \times \text{Hgb(mg/dL)} \times 10}$$

The uptake of oxygen by the lungs can be measured directly using a metabolic cart. Given the unwieldiness, time, and expense, oxygen consumption is often estimated by a formula or nomogram. This simplification can, however, introduce inaccuracies to the calculation, especially in patients with significantly higher or lower metabolic demands than usual (see Troubleshooting: Calculation of Cardiac Output and Cardiac Index).

Factors Affecting Oxygen Consumption

Age
Gender
Hyper or hypothyroidism
Hyper or hypothermia
Exercise
Sepsis

Angiographic Techniques: This method uses the left ventriculogram to estimate stroke volume based on geometric assumptions about the shape of the ventricle. The stroke volume is multiplied by the heart rate, which gives an estimate of cardiac output. This method usually is the least accurate, especially in ventricles that do not hold up to geometric assumptions (Table 7-2).

Troubleshooting

Calculation of Cardiac Output and Cardiac Index

A 56-year-old man:

Height = 180 cm
Weight = 70 kg
Oxygen consumption = 250 mL/min
Arterial O_2 Saturation = 98%
Venous O_2 Saturation = 70%
Hemoglobin = 14 g/dL

$$CO = \frac{oxygen\ consumption\,(mL/min)}{(arterial\ -\ venous\ O_2\ sat)\times 1.36 \times Hgb \times 10}$$

$$CO = \frac{250}{(0.98 - 0.70)(1.36)(14)(10)} = 4.69\ L/min$$

$$BSA = \sqrt{(height\,(cm) \times weight\,(kg)/3600)}$$

$$BSA = \sqrt{(180 \times 70/3600)} = 1.87\ m^2$$

$$CI(L/min/m^2) = CO(L/min)/BSA\,(m^2)$$

$$CI = 4.69/1.87 = 2.51\ L/min/m^2$$

Table **7-2**	Methods for Determining Cardiac Output, and Conditions in Which They Are Most (or Least) Reliable	
Method	**Most reliable**	**Least reliable**
Fick	Low cardiac output	High cardiac output
Thermodilution	High cardiac output	Low cardiac output
		Pulmonic regurgitation
		Tricuspid regurgitation
		Intracardiac shunting
Angiographic	Normal-shaped ventricle	Extensive segmental wall motion abnormalities
		Dilated ventricle
		Aortic regurgitation
		Mitral regurgitation

Left Ventricular Filling Pressures: The left ventricular filling pressures are often estimated by the PCWP. Differentiating the PA pressure from PCWP can sometimes be difficult, especially in the setting of severe mitral regurgitation, but three criteria can be used. **The mean PCWP should be about 10 mm Hg less than the mean PA pressure.** Blood withdrawn from the catheter in the wedged position should have an arterial saturation. Finally, if fluoroscopy is available, the tip is "wedged" when it is lodged and not moving in the distal PA.

The **LVEDP provides the best hemodynamic correlation with the volume status of the heart** and can help guide diuretic and vasodilator therapy. The LVEDP in normal patients is 3 to 12 mm Hg. This parameter may increase with pressure or volume overload and with decreased left ventricular compliance.

Potential Etiologies of Left Ventricular End Diastolic Pressure Elevation

Aortic insufficiency
Mitral regurgitation
Intracardiac shunts
High-output CHF
Hypertension
Hypertrophic cardiomyopathy
Aortic stenosis
Cardiomyopathy—ischemic or nonischemic
Restrictive CM
Infiltrative CM

Vascular Resistance: Resistance is defined as the ratio of the pressure gradient across a vascular bed divided by the flow through that bed. Clinically, the two commonly calculated resistances are the systemic vascular resistance and the pulmonary vascular resistance.

Systemic vascular resistance (SVR) Wood units (mm Hg/L/min) =

$$\frac{\text{mean aortic pressure} - \text{mean RA pressure}}{\text{Qs or CO}}$$

Pulmonary vascular resistance (PVR) Wood units (mm Hg/L/min) =

$$\frac{\text{mean PA pressure} - \text{mean LA pressure}}{\text{Qp or CO}}$$

Units: 80 dynes-sec-cm^5 = 1 Wood unit (or mm Hg/L/min)

In most patients, changes in vascular resistance reflect changes in arteriolar tone or changes in the viscosity of blood (often secondary to anemia). In patients who are hypotensive or in shock, SVR calculations help to differentiate between certain etiologies, and may help guide therapy. For example, a hypotensive patient with a low SVR may have sepsis, while a patient in cardiogenic shock often has hypotension with an elevated SVR.

Acknowledgment

The authors acknowledge the contribution of David Lee to the previous edition of this chapter.

Suggested Reading

Baim DS, ed. *Grossman's Cardiac Catheterization, Angiography, and Intervention.* 7th ed. Philadelphia, PA: Williams & Wilkins; 2005.

Bonow RO, Carabello B, Kanu C, et al. ACC/AHA 2006 guidelines for the management of patients with valvular heart disease: a report of the American College of Cardiology/American Heart Association Task Force on Practice Guidelines *J Am Coll Cardiol.* 2006;48:e1–e148.

Brandfonbrener M, Landowne M, Shock NW. Changes in cardiac output with age. *Circulation.* 1955;12:556.

Fick A. Uber die Messung des Blutguantums in den Herzventrikeln. *Sitz der Physik-Med ges Wurtzberg.* 1870;16.

Gorlin R, Gorlin SG. Hydraulic formula for calculation of the area of the stenotic mitral valve, other cardiac valves, and central circulatory shunts. *Am Heart J.* 1951;41:1.

Hakki AH, Iskandrian AS, Bemis CE, et al. A simplified valve formula for the calculation of stenotic cardiac valve areas. *Circulation.* 1981;63:1050.

Heupler FA. Hemodynamics. Intensive Review of Cardiology Review Course; 2000.

Hurrell DG, Nishimura RA, Higano ST, et al. Value of respiratory changes in left and right ventricular pressures for the diagnosis of constrictive pericarditis. *Circulation.* 1996;93:2007.

Talreja DR, Nishimura RA, Oh JK, et al. Constrictive pericarditis in the modern era: novel criteria for diagnosis in the cardiac catheterization laboratory. *JACC.* 2008;51:315–319.

Kendrick AH, West J, Papouchado M, et al. Direct Fick cardiac output: are assumed values of oxygen consumption acceptable? *Eur Heart J.* 1988;9:337.

Selzer A, Sudrann RB. Reliability of the determination of cardiac output in man by means of the Fick principle. *Circ Res.* 1958;6:485.

Topol EJ, ed. *Textbook of Cardiovascular Medicine.* 2nd ed. Philadelphia, PA: Williams & Wilkins; 2002.

Normal Hemodynamic Values

Flows

Cardiac index (L/min/m^2)	2.6–4.2
Stroke volume index (mL/m^2)	35–55

Pressures (mm Hg)

Aorta/systemic artery	
Peak systolic/end diastolic	100–140/60–90
Mean	70–105
Left ventricle	
Peak systolic/end diastolic	100–140/3–12
Left atrium (pulmonary capillary wedge)	
Mean	1–10
"a" wave	3–15
"v" wave	3–15
Pulmonary artery	
Peak systolic/end diastolic	16–30/0–8
Mean	10–16
Right ventricle	
Peak systolic/end diastolic	16–30/0–8
Right atrium	
Mean	0–8
"a" wave	2–10
"v" wave	2–10

Resistances

Systemic vascular resistance	
Wood units	10–20
Dynes-sec-cm^{-5}	770–1500
Pulmonary vascular resistance	
Wood units	0.25–1.50
Dynes-sec-cm^{-5}	20–120
Oxygen consumption (mL/min/m^2)	110–150
AVO$_2$ difference (mL/dL)	3.0–4.5

AHA/ACC Guidelines for the Management of Patients with Valvular Heart Disease

Recommendations for Cardiac Catheterization in Aortic Stenosis

Indication	Class
1. Coronary angiography before AVR in patients at risk for CAD.	I
2. Assessment of severity of AS in symptomatic patients when AVR is planned or when noninvasive tests are inconclusive or there is a discrepancy with clinical findings regarding severity of AS or need for surgery.	I
3. Coronary angiography is recommended before AVR in patients with AS for whom a pulmonary autograft (Ross procedure) is contemplated and if the origin of the coronary arteries was not identified by noninvasive technique.	I
4. Assessment of severity of AS before AVR when noninvasive tests are adequate and concordant with clinical findings and coronary angiography is not needed.	III
5. Assessment of LV function and severity of AS in asymptomatic patients when noninvasive tests are adequate.	III

Recommendations for Cardiac Catheterization in Chronic Aortic Regurgitation

Indication	Class
1. Coronary angiography before AVR in patients at risk for CAD.	I
2. Assessing severity of regurgitation, LV function, or aortic root size when noninvasive tests are inconclusive or discordant with clinical findings in patients with AR.	I
3. Assessment of LV function and severity of regurgitation before AVR when noninvasive tests are adequate and concordant with clinical findings and coronary angiography is not needed.	III
4. Assessment of LV function and severity of regurgitation in asymptomatic patients when noninvasive tests are adequate.	III

Recommendations for Cardiac Catheterization in Mitral Stenosis

Indication	Class
1. Assess the severity of MS when noninvasive tests are inconclusive or when there is a discrepancy between noninvasive tests and clinical findings regarding the severity of MS.	I
2. Catheterization for hemodynamic evaluation including left ventriculography (to evaluate severity of MR) for patients with MS is indicated when there is a discrepancy between the Doppler-derived mean gradient and valve area.	I
3. Assess hemodynamic response of pulmonary artery and left atrial pressures to exercise when clinical symptoms and resting hemodynamics are discordant.	IIa
4. Assess the cause of severe pulmonary arterial hypertension when out of proportion to severity of MS as determined by noninvasive testing.	IIa
5. Assess mitral valve hemodynamics when 2D and Doppler echocardiography data are concordant with clinical findings.	III

Indications for Cardiac Catheterization in Mitral Regurgitation

Indication	Class
1. Left ventriculography and hemodynamic measurements are indicated when noninvasive tests are inconclusive regarding severity of MR, LV function, or the need for surgery.	I
2. Left ventriculography and hemodynamic measurements are indicated when there is a discrepancy between clinical and noninvasive findings regarding severity of MR.	I
3. Hemodynamic measurements are indicated when pulmonary artery pressure is out of proportion to the severity of MR as assessed by noninvasive testing.	I
4. Coronary angiography is indicated before MV repair or MV replacement in patients at risk for CAD.	I
5. Left ventriculography and hemodynamic measurements are not indicated in patients with MR in whom valve surgery is not contemplated.	III

Adapted from Bonow RO et. al. Circulation 2008;118:e523-e661

CHAPTER 8

Approach to the High-Risk Patient

Daniel J. Cantillon

Adverse events during diagnostic right and left heart catheterization are more likely to occur in high-risk patients (Table 8-1). Procedural indications should be reviewed carefully to justify the increased risk. **An adverse outcome can be avoided by identifying a high-risk patient, implementing preventive measures, and recognizing complications early.**

General preventive measures include correction of any electrolyte abnormalities prior to the procedure; awareness of any pre-existing atrioventricular (AV) nodal block, bundle branch block; or prolongation of the QT on the baseline surface electrocardiogram (EKG) to identify patients at risk for procedural arrhythmias. For patients with renal insufficiency, the amount of contrast dye should be minimized and bi-plane imaging considered when available.

Table 8-1	High-Risk Patients
Left main coronary artery disease	
Severe ventricular dysfunction	
Severe aortic valvular stenosis	
Aortic dissection, aneurysm, or atheroma	
Cardiogenic shock	
Acute coronary syndrome	
Hypertrophic obstructive cardiomyopathy	
Coagulopathy or increased bleeding risk	
Severe pulmonary hypertension	
Acute/chronic kidney disease	
Peripheral vascular disease	

Common Problems in High-Risk Patients

Hypotension: Periprocedureal hypotension may be caused by contrast allergy or contrast-induced vasodilation, vagal response, ischemia, dysrhythmia, hypovolemia, oversedation. It is important to follow a simple algorithm to identify and treat the cause. First, ascertain that hypotension is real and not caused by artifact (i.e., catheter damping or whip). At the same time, identify any changes in rhythm or ST segments. Next concentrate on complications related to the last task performed (Table 8-2). For example, hypotension or dampening of the pressure waveform during attempts to engage the diagnostic catheter into the left main (LM) or right coronary artery should immediately raise concern for severe ostial disease, iatrogenic vasospasm, or coronary dissection. This is especially true when engaging coronary arteries with anomalous origin or in patients

Table **8-2** Troubleshooting Acute Hypotension in the Lab		
Procedural Event Precipitating Acute Hypotension Onset	**Suspected Cause**	**Treatment**
Coronary catheter engagement	Severe ostial disease Vasospasm Iatrogenic dissection	Catheter withdrawal Nitroglycerin 50–200 µg IC PCI or bypass surgery
RCA contrast injection	Vagal stimulation Myocardial ischemia	Avoid over-injection of dye Coronary revascularization
Vascular access (immediate)	Vagal stimulation	Self-limited Atropine 0.5–1 mg IV
Vascular access (delayed)	Bleeding	Volume resuscitation Transfusion Vascular surgery evaluation
Crossing the aortic valve	Aortic dissection Coronary dissection	Emergent surgical correction PCI or bypass surgery
PA catheter or wire manipulation in the RV	RV perforation Cardiac tamponade	Volume resuscitation Pericardiocentesis with drain
PA catheter balloon inflation	Arterial rupture	Volume resuscitation Emergent surgical correction
Transvenous pacing wire	RV perforation	Pericardiocentesis with drain
Immediately post-shock for tachyarrhythmia	Electromechanical dissociation	Fluoroscopy to verify cardiac loss of cardiac motion ACLS protocol for PEA arrest

with heavily calcified and diseased aortas in which a greater degree of catheter manipulation or torque was required.

Hypotension during vascular access is typically vagal-mediated, self-limited and it occurs within minutes of vascular manipulation. Hypotension 30 minutes to 12 hours after vascular access should raise suspicion for retroperitoneal bleeding. Patients commonly complain of unilateral flank or back pain. Hypotension immediately following contrast dye injection of the right coronary artery can also be vagal mediated. Having a patient cough may help clear contrast from the coronary circulation and restore normal heart rate. Typically, the right coronary artery is more likely to spasm when engaged compared to the LM trunk. Both effects are heightened by the presence of flow-limiting coronary lesions, and mitigated by precise catheter control and a smooth engagement technique without allowing the tip of the catheter to become deeply seated.

Hypotension during diagnostic right heart catheterization may be attributable to multiple causes. Forceful advancement of the pulmonary artery (PA) catheter within the right ventricle with the balloon deflated or with the tip deflected away from the outflow tract can result in free wall perforation and tamponade. Similarly, the use of a 0.25-in guidewire when attempting to direct the PA catheter beyond the outflow tract in a dilated and/or dysfunctional ventricle can also easily perforate the right ventricular free wall. An abrupt increase in ventricular ectopy with hypotension while manipulating the catheter or wire in the right ventricle should immediately alert the operator to this possibility. **Aggressive volume expansion is usually the only measure needed to support patients with iatrogenic right ventricular perforation.** Pericardiocentesis with a drain may be necessary in selected cases.

Bradycardia: Transient bradycardia caused by ionic contrast agents or hypervagotonia usually resolves without treatment. **If bradycardia does not resolve spontaneously, treatment with atropine 0.5 to 1 mg IV or more rarely a continuous infusion of dopamine may be required.** A temporary transvenous pacemaker (TVP) may be required in selected cases. A typical presentation requiring temporary pacing support involves a patient with a pre-existing left bundle branch block who develops complete or high-grade AV block while manipulating a catheter in the right ventricle during a right heart catheterization. Prophylactic TVP placement should be considered in these patients. A prophylactic TVP is not indicated for first-degree AV block or Mobitz I second-degree heart block.

General indications for TVP also include symptomatic or hemodynamically significant bradycardia attributable to sinus node dysfunction, high-grade atrioventricular block, and enhanced vagal tone (Table 8-3). Blunt-tipped passive placement (i.e., "contact") pacing wires are most commonly selected as they are easy to use, readily available, and generally atraumatic. **It is important to remember to select the pacemaker wire with the preformed curvature appropriate for the vascular access site.** Passive temporary wires designed for jugular and subclavian access have a smooth terminal curvature (similar to a PA catheter) to allow the wire to be advanced into the right ventricular outflow tract (RVOT) and pulmonary artery and then gently withdrawn into the right ventricle (RV) where counterclock torque will nestle the tip up along the RV floor at or near the apex. Advancing the wire up into the RVOT and the PA outside of the cardiac silhouette is important to ensure the wire has not inadvertently passed into

---

Table 8-3   ACC/AHA Indications for Transvenous Pacemakers in the Setting of Myocardial Infarction

Class I
1. Symptomatic bradycardia
2. Bilateral bundle branch block
3. New or age indeterminate bifascicular block with PR segment prolongation
4. Mobitz type II second-degree AV block

Class IIa
1. New or age indeterminate right bundle branch block (RBBB) with left anterior fascicular block (LAFB) or left posterior fascicular block (LPFB)
2. RBBB with prolonged AV conduction
3. New or age indeterminate left bundle branch block (LBBB)
4. Incessant ventricular tachycardia for overdrive pacing
5. Recurrent sinus pauses greater than 3 seconds not responsive to atropine

Class IIb
1. Bifascicular block of indeterminate age
2. New or age indeterminate isolated RBBB

Class III
1. Prolonged AV conduction
2. Mobitz type I second-degree AV block with normal hemodynamics
3. Accelerated idioventricular rhythm
4. BBB or fascicular block known to exist before myocardial infarction

Adapted from Antman EM, et.al. ACC/AHA Guidelines for the management of patients with ST-Elevation myocardial infarction—Executive summary. Circulation 2004;110:588–636.

the coronary sinus (CS). These wires are not designed for CS pacing. Passive blunt-tipped pacing wires designed for femoral access typically have a J-tipped curvature. Under fluoroscopy, the wire is advanced up into the inferior vena cava (IVC) across the tricuspid valve where the curved tip is directed posteriorly and inferiorly along the RV floor at or near the apex. In patients with right ventricular enlargement, straight or curved balloon-tipped temporary wires are also available.

Active fixation temporary wires are also available and are typically advanced into the appropriate chamber under the guidance of a 6 or 7 Fr. size stiff outer sheath. The outer sheath is directed to the desired location under fluoroscopy approximately 0.5 to 1 cm away from the wall. The wire is then advanced beyond the sheath to the wall and torqued clockwise to screw it into place. Gently retracting the outer sheath and testing capture thresholds verifies appropriate fixation. Active fixation wires are particularly helpful for atrial pacing, when getting a stable position with good capture is often difficult with the blunt-tipped passive wires. The outer sheath must be carefully advanced and never allowed to tent the myocardium.

Regardless of wire selection, pacing output should be initiated under fluoroscopy. Sudden diaphragmatic movements tracking pacemaker spikes indicate diaphragmatic pacing requiring lead repositioning. The capture threshold, defined as the lowest current necessary for capture, should be established. Output is generally started at 5 mA and slowly decreased until capture is lost. Once the capture threshold is obtained (ideally less than 1 mA), the output is set to two to three times the capture threshold as a safety margin. Sensing thresholds are then tested by setting the pacing rate 10 to 20 beats below the intrinsic rate with the pacemaker in its most sensitive setting (lowest mV recognition available). The sensitivity is then gradually increased until asynchronous pacing occurs. This is the point at which the device can no longer detect the native QRS complex because the threshold has been set higher than the amplitude of the native complex. The pacemaker is then programmed to sense at 50% of the sensing threshold as a safety margin.

The most common complications of TVP insertion include vascular or myocardial rupture or damage, cardiac tamponade, induction of cardiac arrhythmias, pneumothorax, and bleeding complications at the access site.

Tachycardia: Registry data suggests that ventricular tachycardia or fibrillation complicates 0.4% of all diagnostic catheterizations. If a tachyarrhyhmia causes hemodynamic compromise, ACLS (advanced cardiac life support) protocols should be initiated promptly. "Cough CPR (cardiopulmonary resuscitation)" may help the patient maintain consciousness during a ventricular arrhythmia by accelerating venous return and augmenting cardiac output. However, early defibrillation and initiation of antiarrhythmic medications, such as amiodarone 150 to 300 mg and/or lidocaine 1 mg/kg or empirically 100 mg, are recommended whenever a patient develops malignant ventricular tachycardia. Continuous infusions of these medications after the loading dose are generally indicated to prevent recurrent arrhythmias.

Atrial fibrillation (AF) with ventricular response can pose a problem during the procedure. Hemodynamic instability merits cardioversion under ACLS protocol. However, the risk of embolic stroke favors rate control when possible when the duration of AF is greater than 48 hours or uncertain. Traditional AV nodal agents such as β-blocker and calcium channel blockers are the first-line drugs. However, digoxin, while an older drug, is often effective and a largely forgotten therapy in the cath lab. In appropriately selected patients, a loading dose of 0.5 mg IV may slow the ventricular response within 30 minutes and provide a durable response for the duration of the procedure. A full loading dose of digoxin is generally 1 g over 24 hours. Caution is advised in patients with potassium levels outside the range of normal or in patients with renal dysfunction.

Airway Compromise/Respiratory Failure: Most diagnostic heart catheterizations are performed under conscious sedation rather than general anesthesia. **Hence, any airway compromise or respiratory failure during the procedure requires prompt attention as progressive hypoxemia, hypercapnea, and acidemia may lower the threshold for ventricular arrhythmias and increase the risk of cardiac arrest.**

A focused preprocedural physical examination of the patient verifies adequate respiratory/pulmonary status to tolerate laying flat for the duration of the procedure and candidacy for conscious sedation. Patients with acutely decompensated heart failure are often better served having an elective diagnostic catheterization after adequate diuresis and medical optimization. Additionally, it is good practice to assess the patient's neck habitus and visualize the uvula, as well as asking about any difficulty with endotracheal intubation in the past to identify patients in whom obtaining an emergent airway might become a problem. A Mallampati airway score is used routinely in some cath labs to identify potentially difficult tracheal intubations. A Mallampati classification is an estimate of the tongue size relative to the oral cavity.

When respiratory failure does occur in the lab, it is important to rapidly discriminate procedural iatrogenic causes (such as oversedation with opiates and benzodiazepines), and patient factors (intrinsic pulmonary disease, acutely decompensated failure, etc.). The latter may prompt endotracheal intubation, while the former can be rapidly reversed by administering naloxone 0.4 mg, an opiate receptor antagonist.

Specific High-Risk Patient Scenarios

Acute Coronary Syndrome (ACS): In all patients with ACS, especially those with ST segment elevation myocardial infarction, the goal is to quickly and accurately assess all major epicardial vessels in at least two orthogonal views while rapidly identifying the culprit lesion(s) so that either percutaneous or surgical revascularization may proceed. These patients are at high risk of life-threatening arrhythmias, cardiogenic shock, and death. Use of anticoagulants and anti-platelet medications places these patients at higher risk of bleeding and vascular complications.

There are important strategic considerations for the diagnostic procedure in high-risk ACS patients. In the setting of acute STEMI (ST-segment elevation myocardial infarction), some operators elect to begin coronary angiography by imaging the opposite vessel of the ECG-predicted acute infarct artery using a diagnostic catheter, and then proceed with angiography of the infarct vessel using a guide catheter to allow a rapid transition to percutaneous intervention. The major advantage is obviating the time spent exchanging a diagnostic catheter for a guide catheter to re-engage the infarct vessel. This strategy is particularly useful when patients with triple vessel disease or pre-existing critical stenosis in one major epicardial vessel develop coronary plaque rupture and acute STEMI in the opposite artery. By starting in the noninfarct artery, one can identify a lesion that might alter the patient's management. For example, critical LM or proximal LAD disease in a patient with an acute RCA infarct might prompt a decision to refer for emergent coronary artery bypass grafting or at least the prophylactic placement of an intra-aortic balloon pump before beginning percutaneous intervention on the infarct-related RCA.

Left Main Trunk Coronary Artery Disease: According to the Society for Cardiac Angiography and Interventions, patients with LM disease have a twofold greater risk of complications from cardiac catheterization. Angiography of a patient with severe LM stenosis (Figure 8-1) may produce profound hypotension, thereby potentiating myocardial ischemia. **LM disease should be suspected in patients with a markedly positive stress test (LV, left ventricle, dilation on stress and/or lung uptake of sestamibi), ischemic ECG changes in a large, anterior distribution, or in patients presenting with ACS with associated heart failure.** Often, the first clue suggesting LM stenosis is dampening of the catheter upon engagement of the LM ostium (Figure 8-2). If this occurs, the catheter should be promptly removed and carefully re-engaged approaching the LM from a slightly different angle. If dampening recurs and is not rectified with careful catheter manipulation, then the catheter should be removed and a subselective injection performed. Injection

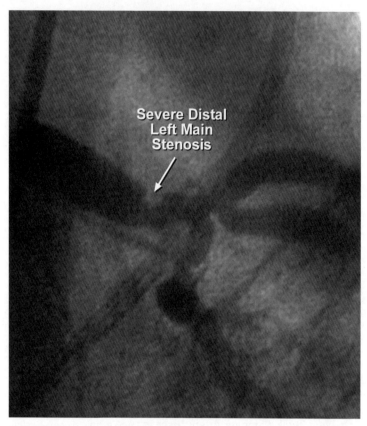

Figure **8-1** Angiogram demonstrating a severe distal LM trunk stenosis *(arrow)*.

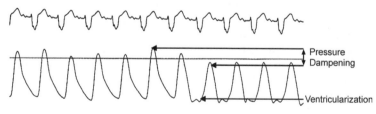

Figure **8-2** Pressure dampening and ventricularization upon catheter engagement of the left main (LM) trunk. Waveform alterations seen upon catheter engagement of a severe LM trunk stenosis. Clues to LM stenosis include a pressure gradient (dampening) and ventricularization of the pressure waveform.

into the left CS will often be enough to unmask severe disease. Subsequent injections should be made with nonionic contrast and limited to revealing targets for bypass grafts. In most cases the entire study of the left system can be limited to two subselective injections, consisting of a straight PA cranial (left anterior descending artery view) and an RAO caudal angulated view (left circumflex artery view).

Aortic Dissection or Aneurysm: The rationale for coronary angiography prior to surgical correction of aortic dissection is to identify severe coronary lesions that should be grafted at the time of open heart surgery. **However, there are data suggesting that coronary angiography in patients with type A aortic dissection does not improve in-hospital mortality.** Cardiac CT (computed tomography) angiography is emerging as a noninvasive substitute for invasive angiography in patients with aortic disease and a low to intermediate probability for coronary artery disease. Nonetheless, conventional coronary angiography remains the mainstay of preoperative evaluation of patients with aortic pathology.

Catheter selection and techniques utilized should be made with knowledge of the specific aortic anatomy and pathology. For patients with ascending aortic aneurysms, the use of longer tipped catheters such as the JL5 or JL6 may be necessary to reach the LM trunk ostium. Use of the multipurpose catheter may be necessary to reach the right coronary ostium due to effacement of the aortic root. Additionally, choosing the appropriate vascular access site can help avoid engaging the false aortic lumen in the case of aortic dissection or avoiding diseased segments in the case of aneurysmal disease. For example, obtaining right radial or brachial access should be considered in patients with aortic dissection sparing the ascending aorta but involving the arch beyond the innominate artery or the proximal descending aorta. When traversing dissected aorta is unavoidable, using soft-tipped exchange-length wires and longer sheath minimizes the risk of aortic trauma and keeps catheters inside the true lumen. When in doubt, gentle nonselective contrast injections in orthogonal views with cine angiography can help identify the coronary ostia, as well as the catheter tip location with respect to the false lumen. This can help the operator select catheters most appropriate to safely engage the ostium. The true lumen usually has brisk pulsatile flow, whereas flow within the false lumen appears static and often fails to clear rapidly. Only nonselective views of the coronary arteries may be obtainable in some cases.

Aortic Stenosis: **The goals of cardiac catheterization in patient with aortic stenosis (AS) are to confirm the diagnosis of outflow obstruction, localize the obstruction (subvalvular, valvular, or**

supravalvular), estimate the severity of the stenosis, estimate the left ventricular function, and evaluate the coronary circulation. Patients with AS are more likely to have aortic root dilation, especially in the setting of a bicuspid aortic valve, which may require alternate catheter selection for coronary angiography. Complications of cardiac catheterization in patients with AS include dysrhythmias, myocardial perforation, cardiac tamponade, stroke, myocardial infarction, and death. **The aortic valve does not need to be crossed if valve surgery is planned on the basis of the noninvasive assessment.**

Transient hypotension and/or bradycardia may be life threatening in patients with critical AS. In cases of profound and protracted hypotension, intra-aortic balloon pump (IABP) counterpulsation may serve as a "bridge" to definitive therapy. If hypotension occurs while trying to cross the valve, perforation of the CS with resultant tamponade should be suspected. In such cases, rapid surgical intervention is necessary.

Ventricular arrhythmias are life threatening in patients with severe AS because intravenous medications tend not to circulate well in the setting of severe outflow obstruction. **If asystolic or pulseless electrical activity (PEA) arrest occurs in a patient with critical AS, ACLS protocol should be initiated, and intracardiac epinephrine (5 mg) should be given early in the resuscitative effort.**

Cardiogenic Shock: Patients presenting to the catheterization lab in cardiogenic shock are at very high risk for morbidity and mortality during catheterization. Cardiogenic shock occurs in 5% to 15% of patients with an acute myocardial infarction. In the GUSTO I trial, patients presenting in cardiogenic shock accounted for 58% of the mortality in the entire trial. The overriding goal of cardiac catheterization in patients with cardiogenic shock is to rapidly identify the coronary lesion(s) responsible. Most operators will place an IABP prior to angiography in order to minimize the risk of further hemodynamic collapse. Patients with cardiogenic shock may benefit from routine placement of a pulmonary artery (Swan-Ganz) catheter for guided therapy following the procedure in the ICU (intensive care unit).

Indications and contraindications of IABP placement are listed in Table 8-4. When first introduced in 1962, IABPs were surgically placed. Beginning in 1980, however, the percutaneous approach via the femoral artery replaced the surgical approach as the primary means of insertion. **Balloon size is selected based on the patient's height. Most patients receive a 40-cc balloon. Patients shorter than 64 in or taller than 72 in require smaller (34 cc) or larger (50 cc) balloons, respectively.** The IABP can be inserted either through a sheath (8 or 9.5 Fr.) or via a sheathless technique.

Table **8-4**	Indications and Contraindications to IABP Placement
Indications	**Contraindications**
Cardiogenic shock	Moderate aortic insufficiency (>2+)
Severe mitral regurgitation	Abdominal aortic aneurysm
Decompensated aortic stenosis	Aortic dissection
Ventricular septal defect	Bilateral lower extremity PVD
Refractory ischemia	Significant arteriovenous shunts
High-risk PCI	Severe coagulopathy
Bridge to definitive therapy	Sepsis
	No planned definitive therapy

After vascular access has been obtained, the IABP is inserted into the descending thoracic aorta over a guidewire. Fluoroscopic guidance is essential to achieve optimal placement in the aorta. The proximal radiopaque tip should be located just below the subclavian artery or at the level of the carina (Figure 8-3), and the distal end should be above the renal arteries (usually at the level of L1–L2) and completely out of the sheath. The central lumen is aspirated and flushed with heparinized saline and connected to a pressure transducer. The balloon is then connected to the pump and filled to half volume. Adequate filling and location should be confirmed by fluoroscopy. Once location is confirmed, the IABP is filled completely and then secured with sutures. Patients are routinely placed on systemic anticoagulation to prevent potential thromboembolic complications resulting from an indwelling intravascular device. However, manufacturers of IABPs indicate that systemic anticoagulation is optional.

Optimal adjustment of the timing and triggers results in maximum hemodynamic effects (Figure 8-4). Timing of inflation should correlate with the onset of diastole. To properly adjust timing of inflation, the IABP should be placed on an inflation ratio of 1:2 to observe augmented and unaugmented beats. The central pressure waveform is used to guide proper timing. Ideally, the balloon should inflate with the closure of the aortic valve, identified by the dicrotic notch of the central pressure waveform tracing. Deflation should occur with aortic valve opening, which can be timed with the onset of the R wave by ECG tracing. When timed appropriately, the central aortic waveform should have an augmentation pressure greater than the systolic pressure, and a post-deflation pressure 10 to 15 mm Hg below the unaugmented diastolic blood pressure.

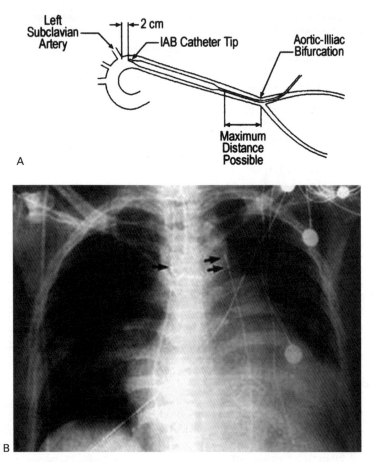

Figure **8-3** **Optimal positioning of the intra-aortic balloon pump.**
A) Diagram demonstrating the optimal positioning of the IABP approximately 2 cm distal to the left subclavian artery. **B)** The radio-opaque tip of the IABP is located approximately 2 cm cranial to the left mainstem bronchus at the level of the carina *(double arrowheads).*

After IABP insertion, patients should have daily checks of hemoglobin, hematocrit, platelet count, white blood cell count, renal function, and a chest x-ray for placement. Meticulous attention to peripheral pulses and access site is of paramount importance in detecting early vascular complications.

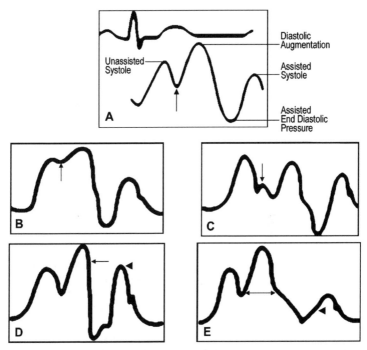

Figure **8-4   Timing of IABP inflation and deflation. A)** Correct timing: With correct timing of IABP inflation and deflation an augmentation of diastolic and systolic blood pressures is seen. Inflation occurs at the onset of diastole *(arrow)* and deflation should occur prior to the onset of systole *(arrowhead)*, resulting in decreased aortic end diastolic and systolic pressures. **B)** Premature inflation: Inflation of IABP prior to dicrotic notch *(arrow)*. This may result in premature aortic valve closure, increased LV wall stress, aortic regurgitation, and increased myocardial oxygen demand. **C)** Delayed inflation: Inflation of IABP following the dicrotic notch *(arrow)* may result in inadequate accentuation of coronary perfusion. **D)** Premature deflation: Observed as a precipitous drop in the pressure waveform following diastolic augmentation *(arrow)*. Other observations include a suboptimal diastolic augmentation and an assisted systole that is equal or greater than the unassisted systole *(arrowhead)*. This may result in suboptimal afterload reduction and increased myocardial oxygen demand. **E)** Delayed deflation: Observed as an assisted end diastolic pressure equal to or greater than the unassisted end diastolic pressure, a prolonged rate of rise of the assisted systole *(arrowhead)*, and a widened diastolic augmentation *(double arrow)*. A lack of afterload reduction and an increase in myocardial oxygen demand occur.

Table **8-5**	Common Complications Associated with IABP Counterpulsation
Vascular **(6–25%[a])**	**Nonvascular** **(4–15%[a])**
Hematoma formation	Sepsis
Arterial dissection	Thrombocytopenia
Vascular laceration	Hemolysis
Limb ischemia	Groin infection
Thromboembolic complications	Peripheral neuropathy
Renal ischemia	
Spinal cord ischemia	

[a]Incidence.

Complications can be divided into vascular and nonvascular complications (Table 8-5). Vascular complications occur in 6% to 25% of cases. Specific complications include limb ischemia, arterial dissection, vascular laceration (requiring surgical repair), and major hemorrhage.

Pulmonary Hypertension: Indications for cardiac catheterization in patients with pulmonary hypertension include determination of cause, assessment of severity, reversibility, quantification of intracardiac shunts, and pulmonary angiography. During any right heart catheterization, the sudden onset of shortness of breath or hypoxemia and hypotension may indicate pneumothorax during jugular or subclavian access, pulmonary embolus, or cardiac perforation. In general, inflation of the balloon into a pulmonary capillary wedge position is safe, well tolerated and provides valuable diagnostic information. However, patients with severe pulmonary arterial hypertension are at increased risk of PA rupture. Hypotension in a patient with spontaneous cough (especially hemoptysis) after prolonged inflation of the balloon in the pulmonary capillary wedge position should raise the concern for PA rupture, especially in a patient with underlying severe pulmonary arterial hypertension. Aggressive volume expansion and surgical evaluation are warranted.

Increased Bleeding Risk: Patients with thrombocytopenia or coagulopathy are at increased risk for bleeding complications from diagnostic catheterization (i.e., hematoma or retroperitoneal bleed). The precise threshold at which point a cardiac catheterization becomes contraindicated is somewhat controversial and depends on the indication for the study. Many centers use a platelet count of less than 50,000 or an international normalized ratio (INR) of greater than 2.0. However, it is inappropriate to delay taking a patient to the lab coming through the emergency department with an acute ST elevation myocardial infarction by waiting on an INR or platelet level to return. For patients with INR >2.0, there are data to suggest that manual sheath removal and pressure hemostasis are preferred to reduce bleeding complications, or suturing the sheath in place for removal after coagulopathy reversal. For patients with increased bleeding risk, vascular access trauma can be minimized by using commercially available micropuncture kits with smaller needles, wires, and sheaths that can be upsized to more traditional sheath sizes to accommodate diagnostic catheters. Additionally, venous puncture of the internal jugular vein for right heart catheterization can be performed under direct ultrasound guidance when bleeding risk is a concern.

When a retroperitoneal bleed is suspected, a noncontrast CT scan of the abdomen and pelvis with extension of axial imaging to mid-thigh is the best modality to establish the diagnosis. Vascular surgical consultation may be necessary; however, the majority of these events are managed conservatively with volume resuscitation, hemodynamic monitoring in an ICU with serial measurements of hemoglobin or hematocrit. Prompt reversal of coagulatopathy with transfusion of frozen plasma and/or platelets is often necessary, especially in patients with life-threatening bleeds.

Acknowledgments

The author acknowledges the contribution to this chapter of Michael R. Tamberella, MD, and A. Michael Lincoff, MD, from the previous version of this book.

Suggested Reading

Bertrand ME. Identification of intervention patients at increased risk. *Am Heart J.* 1995;130:647–650.

Boehrer JD, Lange RA, Willard JE, et al. Markedly increased periprocedure mortality of cardiac catheterization in patients with severe narrowing of the left main coronary artery. *Am J Cardiol.* 1992;70:1388–1390.

Penn MS, Smedira N, Lytle B, et al. Does coronary angiography before emergency aortic surgery affect in-hospital mortality? *J Am Coll Cardiol.* 2000;35:889–894.

CHAPTER 9

Hemostatic Devices

James E. Harvey and A. Michael Lincoff

Obtaining hemostasis in patients after cardiovascular catheterization is a critical component of the procedure. When the novel technique for percutaneous endovascular access was introduced by Seldinger over 50 years ago, his reported method for achieving hemostasis included "20 to 30 minutes of hand-held pressure after catheter removal followed by overnight bed rest." Since then, manual pressure or mechanical compression has remained the gold standard for achieving postprocedural hemostasis following femoral artery puncture. However, with the increase in coronary and peripheral vascular procedures over the past two decades has come a demand for more efficient and cost-effective methods of achieving hemostasis. This has led to the development of many types of vascular closure devices (VCDs) designed to increase patient comfort while maintaining safety and ease-of-use. These devices offer the advantages of early sheath removal, early ambulation, and early hospital discharge, as well as allow for uninterrupted anticoagulation when needed. In addition to manual compression or mechanical compression devices (including mechanical clamp devices and hemostatic pads), the currently available VCDs fall into three major categories: collagen-based biosealant, percutaneous suture based, and staples and clips, with minimal variation in cost between the devices ($175 to $190 at our institution).

Devices

Manual Compression: Despite many available VCDs on the market, manual pressure remains a fundamental component of arteriotomy management because of its low cost, good safety profile (complication rate of 0.23% following diagnostic catheterization in large series and >50 years experience), short learning curve, and ability to be employed despite femoral artery dissection, significant peripheral vascular disease, or a "low stick." Limitations of this technique include the length of time needed before ambulation, prolonged hospitalization time, need for trained personnel, patient discomfort, staff fatigue, and slowing of the catheterization laboratory workflow. For patients following percutaneous coronary intervention (PCI) or in those who have been on anticoagulation with heparin, manual compression can be safely performed once the activated clotting time (ACT) is less than 180 seconds or the activated partial thromboplastin time (aPTT) is less than 50 seconds.

When removing the sheath, gentle pressure is applied over the skin puncture site being careful not to crush the sheath and "strip" clot into the femoral artery. Manual pressure is then held directly above the arteriotomy at a point approximately 1.5 cm cephalad to the skin puncture site. **Pressure should be held for approximately 3 minutes per French size for arterial punctures and 2 minutes per French size for venous punctures and can be gradually reduced over that time** (i.e., after a 6-Fr. arterial sheath removal, hold full pressure for 5 minutes, then 75% pressure for 5 minutes, then 50% pressure for 5 minutes, then 25% pressure for 3 to 5 minutes). The pedal pulses should be checked every few minutes during femoral artery compression. If the pedal pulses are absent during femoral artery compression, the pressure should be intermittently reduced to allow perfusion to the distal lower extremity. Keep in mind that this is only an estimate and that patients with a mildly elevated ACT or those receiving antiplatelet therapy (i.e., aspirin, clopidogrel, prasugrel, etc.) may need an additional 10 to 15 minutes of manual pressure to achieve hemostasis. Low-risk patients should remain supine for 2 to 3 hours (0.5 hours per French size) after hemostasis, especially when a small diameter catheter is used (≤5 Fr.); high-risk patients should remain supine for 4 to 6 hours after hemostasis. One study involving low-risk patients (5-Fr. sheath, diagnostic catheterization only, no anticoagulation) who received 10 to 15 minutes of manual compression followed by 1 hour of bed rest and 1 hour of observation reported a minor complication rate of 3.3% and a major complication rate of 0.1%. The major complication of manual compression is pseudoaneurysm that results from poor hemostasis (pressure).

Hemostatic Pads: Hemostatic pads (D-Stat Dry, SyvekPatch, Chito-Seal) are small pieces of gauze or other material that are impregnated with a procoagulant mixture that causes local vasoconstriction and potentiates clot formation. Used in conjunction with manual compression, the patch is applied topically over the puncture site after sheath removal and remotely activates the coagulation cascade from the skin surface. Coagulation cascade activation is potentiated down the sheath tract to the arterial wall. The benefits of patches include decreased time to hemostasis, reduced time to ambulation, no insertion of foreign material into the body, and immediate repeat arterial puncture if necessary. Other advantages include shortened hospitalization and a low incidence of major vascular complications (0.1%).

D-Stat Dry hemostatic bandage (Vascular Solutions, Inc., Minneapolis, MN) is a nonwoven gauze patch that is coated with thrombin that potentiates the coagulation cascade by directly converting fibrinogen to fibrin. It is used as an adjunct to manual compression and is indicated to reduce the time to hemostasis in patients undergoing diagnostic endovascular procedures utilizing 4- to 6-Fr. sheaths. A recent study of 367 patients looked at the use of D-Stat Dry versus manual compression alone and found that use of D-Stat Dry resulted in a significant reduction in time to hemostasis (7.8 vs. 13.0 min; $p = 0.001$) with no significant difference in major or minor complications. The D-Stat Dry patch is directly applied over the skin puncture site and manually compressed for a minimum of 6 minutes (for low-risk normotensive patients not anticoagulated) to 10 minutes (anticoagulated, hypertensive, large sheath size) or until hemostasis is achieved. ACT should be less than 180 seconds or in accordance with the local institutional guidelines. Not anticoagulated patients should not ambulate for 1.5 (4 Fr.) to 2.5 (6 Fr.) hours; anticoagulated patients should not ambulate for 2 to 4 hours. D-Stat Dry is contraindicated in patients with known sensitivity to bovine-derived materials.

SyvekPatch (Marine Polymer Technologies, Inc., Danvers, MA) is made of poly-*N*-acetyl glucosamine (p-GlcNAc), which causes local vasoconstriction and potentiates clot formation. This small patch should be applied directly over the arterial puncture site and manually compressed for 10 minutes following sheath extraction. ACT should be less than 300 seconds. Patients are required to lie supine for 2 hours after the patch has been held in place. An uncontrolled study of 200 patients who underwent diagnostic coronary angiography with a 6-Fr. catheter evaluated the use of the SyvekPatch as an adjunct to manual pressure followed by 1 hour of bed rest reported no major and only 2% minor adverse events, all of which were successfully managed with additional 1 to 2 hours of bed rest.

Mechanical Compression: Mechanical compression involves the use of a C-arm clamp, sandbags, or a pneumatic compression device (FemStop). The C-arm clamp is a device with a flat base and a horizontal arm that extends over the base and angles down at a 90° angle to apply pressure to the femoral artery. The tip of the device consists of a metal or plastic disk, which is placed directly over the arterial puncture site for approximately 20 to 30 minutes. The FemStop applies direct

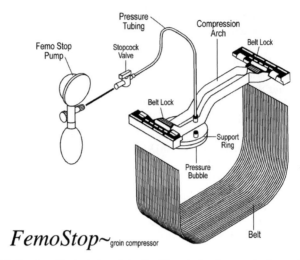

$Femo Stop$~groin compressor

Figure **9-1**   Graphic depiction of the FemStop device for vascular hemostasis. This type of mechanical compression device places a transparent plastic bubble over the arterial puncture site and secures it with a plastic arch and belt wrapped around the patient. (Courtesy of RADI Medical Systems, Inc., Reading, MA.)

pneumatic pressure over the femoral artery to tamponade bleeding. A transparent plastic bubble is placed over the arterial puncture site and secured with a plastic arch and belt wrapped around the patient (Figure 9-1).

A recent study that compared manual to mechanical compression demonstrated that time to hemostasis was approximately 33% shorter with manual compression. Studies done in the 1970s and 1980s noted that there were no significant differences in rates of vascular complications between manual and mechanical compression techniques. Although mechanical compression devices provide a hands-free approach, they do not eliminate the need for staff supervision during the period of compression.

Collagen-based Biosealant Devices: Collagen-based biosealant VCDs utilize bovine collagen-based products to facilitate clot formation. These VCDs augment hemostasis via two mechanisms: (1) the device deploys a collagen mass that expands after deployment and mechanically seals the arterial wall and sheath tract and (2) it provides additional collagen to the arterial wall defect promoting platelet adherence, activation, and aggregation.

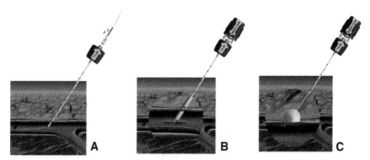

Figure **9-2** **The Angio-Seal closure device. A)** Carrier sheath inserted over a guidewire into vascular lumen. Blood flow through vessel locator verifies correct intravascular positioning. **B)** Device inserted into artery with anchor exposed. Note arrow-to-arrow design of this device ensures correct insertion. **C)** Collagen plug and anchor "sandwich" the arteriotomy site with the use of the tamper tube.

Collagen-based VCDs are generally used in patients who are un-likely to require immediate repeat arterial access. Due to the expansive collagen product, it may be difficult to reaccess the artery close to the previous puncture site and it is usually recommended to wait 90 days until repeat puncture at the same site is attempted. Collagen-based devices should only be used when arterial access was obtained with a single anterior puncture of the common femoral artery. Several different models of colla-gen-based VCDs are commercially available; the three most common are Angio-Seal, DuettPro, and VasoSeal.

Angio-Seal (St. Jude Medical, St. Paul, Minn) is a popular collagen-based VCD that involves placing a collagen plug directly over an intravascular anchoring system. First, a carrier sheath is exchanged for the femoral artery sheath (Figure 9-2). Once inserted, the intravascular an-chor protrudes from the end of the carrier into the femoral artery. The sheath and carrier are then removed, which pulls the intravascular anchor against the inside of the arterial wall. Tension is applied to the connecting suture, advancing the collagen plug down onto the outside of the arterial wall defect. **The patient is required to remain in the supine position for 2 hours after the Angio-Seal has been deployed. Repeat arterial puncture should not be performed for a period of 90 days.** With re-gards to safety and efficacy, a randomized trial comparing the Angio-Seal to manual pressure showed that time to hemostasis following angiogra-phy was significantly shorter in the Angio-Seal group (2.5 minutes) com-pared with manual pressure (15.3 minutes). This study also demonstrated

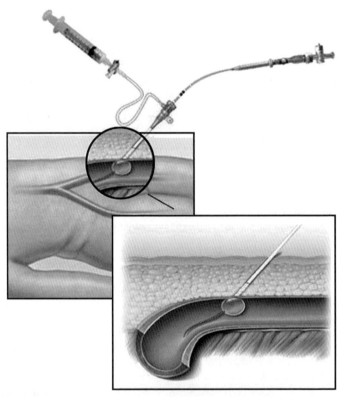

Figure **9-3**   The Duett closure device. Balloon-positioning catheter within the femoral artery and attached syringe of procoagulant mixture. Balloon tamponade of arteriotomy while procoagulant is injected into tissue surrounding puncture site (inset).

significantly fewer complications, such as bleeding and/or hematoma formation, for Angio-Seal patients receiving heparin. In general, the Angio-Seal device affords rapid deployment, earlier hospital discharge, and improved patient comfort following cardiac catheterization. It has also been used successfully used in radial, carotid, and subclavian arterial puncture sites, venous puncture sites, and even right ventricular perforation. It has the lowest reported vascular complication rates of all closure devices.

The **DuettPro** sealing device (Vascular Solutions, Minneapolis, MN) is a collagen-based VCD that utilizes a 7-mm balloon attached to a 3-Fr. catheter to inject a procoagulant mixture of collagen and thrombin (Figure 9-3). The device is advanced through the existing femoral sheath into the arterial lumen, the mounted balloon is inflated in the artery, and then the entire device is gently retracted until the balloon abuts the arteriotomy puncture site. The mixture of collagen and thrombin is injected to the tissue surrounding the arterial puncture site. Thrombin in the presence of collagen converts fibrinogen to fibrin and accelerates the coagulation cascade. The sheath is removed, the balloon is deflated, and manual pressure is applied for 2 minutes. **Patients are required to remain in the supine position for approximately 2 hours** to promote adequate hemostasis and reduce the risk of complications. **Unlike the Angio-Seal device, there is no contraindication to immediate repuncture with the Duett device.** One serious potential complication of the Duett device is the inadvertent injection of the procoagulant collagen–thrombin mixture into the artery. A large study comparing the Duett device to manual pressure showed that the times to hemostasis and ambulation were significantly lower with the Duett device, but the incidence of major vascular complications was higher.

The **VasoSeal** hemostatic devices (VasoSeal Elite and VasoSeal ES; Datascope, Montvale, NJ) are collagen-based VCDs that utilize a purified collagen plug to accentuate hemostasis. To deploy these devices, a dilator and a sheath are collectively advanced over a guidewire to the surface of the femoral artery (Figure 9-4). The dilator is removed and the collagen plug is advanced through the sheath into the vascular access track. **Following placement of the device, patients are kept supine for 2 hours.** This device is similar to the Angio-Seal device in that it delivers a collagen plug into the skin tract; however, there is no intraluminal component remaining after the device is deployed. In patients undergoing coronary angiography, the Vasoseal device had mean times to hemostasis and ambulation of 18 minutes and 110 minutes,

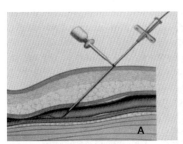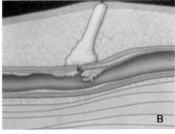

Figure **9-4   The VasoSeal closure device. A)** Dilator advanced over guidewire to previously demarcated depth at surface of femoral artery. **B)** Collagen injected over arteriotomy site while simultaneously withdrawing delivery apparatus resulting in vascular hemostasis.

respectively; however, an increase in vascular complications following PCI has been noted.

A prospective randomized controlled trial directly compared the safety and efficacy of Angio-Seal, Duett, and VasoSeal ES and found the devices to have similar rates of successful deployment and complication. Of note, in the diagnostic arm of this study, the Angio-Seal device did require a longer time to achieve hemostasis; however, it also resulted in earlier ambulation ($p = 0.0001$). A second randomized trial published in the same year directly compared Angio-Seal and VasoSeal in patients undergoing diagnostic coronary angiography and angioplasty. No statistically significant difference was found in time to hemostasis, time to ambulation, device failure, or postprocedural complications. It is important to realize that all of these models of VCDs have been modified by the manufacturer since these studies were published and no randomized controlled trials directly comparing the currently marketed devices exist.

Percutaneous Suture Devices: Percutaneous suture VCDs deploy a pair of needles at the arteriotomy site and enable a knot to be thrown and tied at the level of the artery wall. Arterial closure is usually instant and immediate repuncture is possible. **These devices are advantageous for patients with large arterial punctures, procedures needing uninterrupted anticoagulation, or whenever repeat arterial access is anticipated.** A common limitation of percutaneous suture VCDs is that most are complex and require significant operator training before he/she is competent in its use. Common commercially available percutaneous suture VCDs include the Perclose devices (Proglide and Prostar XL), SuperStitch, and X-Press.

Perclose Proglide (Abbott Vascular, Abbott Labs, IL) is a popular and well-established single suture VCD that is indicated to close arteriotomy sites following percutaneous diagnostic and interventional procedures using a 5-Fr. to 8-Fr. system. Perclose also makes a **Prostar XL** device designed for larger sheath sizes (6.5 to 10 Fr.) that utilizes a four-needle, bisuture system that ties and secures two sutures at the arteriotomy site. However, for larger catheter–based procedures (>8 Fr.), many practitioners simply place two Proglide devices at a perpendicular angle to each other prior to dilating the arteriotomy to a sheath size greater than that indicated for the single suture device ("preclose" technique). Using this technique, the sutures are in place prior to removal of the larger catheter and the arteriotomy can be closed with two sutures following completion of the procedure.

To deploy, the Perclose devices are inserted over a 0.038-in. wire (or smaller) after sheath removal and advanced until blood returns from

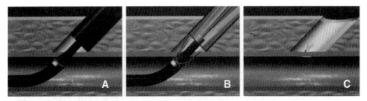

Figure **9-5   The Perclose closure device. A)** Perclose system within femoral artery. **B)** Deployment of suture. **C)** Hemostasis achieved with tamping of knot down to arteriotomy.

a marker lumen (Figure 9-5). The lever on the device handle is raised thereby deploying the footplate in the vessel lumen. The device is withdrawn until the footplate is against the intraluminal wall, and then the plunger is depressed, delivering two needles through the artery wall to the footplate. The needles attach to the suture and the plunger is withdrawn, thereby pulling the suture out through the center of the device. The footplate is retracted and the device is partially pulled out allowing a knot pusher to be inserted onto the exposed suture and advance the pre-tied knot to the level of the arteriotomy. The device is removed and the suture/knot are tightened; hemostatis is usually instant. **Following the placement of the percutaneous suture, patients are required to remain in the supine position for 1 to 2 hours.**

SuperStitch (Sutura, Inc., Fountain Valley, CA) is a relatively new percutaneous suture device that utilizes a nonabsorbable monofilament polypropylene suture to close the arteriotomy site (Figure 9-6). The device has a specially designed tip that allows it to be used in antegrade procedures and to be advanced into the lumen without wire guidance. It is indicated for use after percutaneous endovascular procedures using a 6- to 8-Fr. catheter system. Unlike the other percutaneous suture–mediated devices, SuperStitch has a three-button handle specially designed for ease-

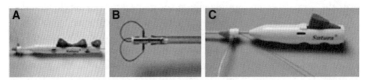

Figure **9-6   A)** SuperStitch device. **B)** Tip of device. **C)** Kwiknot. (Images provided courtesy of Sutura Inc.)

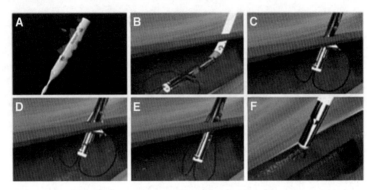

Figure **9-7** **Deployment of SuperStitch Device. A)** The device is advanced through an existing sheath. The first button is depressed. **B)** This opens out the "arms". **C)** The device is retracted against the vessel wall. **D)** Button number 2 is depressed, which deploys the needles. **E)** Button number 3 closes the "arms". The needles retract and draw the sutures out of the vessel. **F)** The knot can be tied manually or by using the Kwiknot device. The Kwiknot ties and cuts the suture close to the vessel wall. (Images provided courtesy of Sutura Inc.)

of-use; the manufacturer states that deploying the device is "as simple as 1-2-3." Device deployment is described in Figure 9-7. In an uncontrolled, prospective study of 150 patients who underwent femoral artery closure with the SuperStitch device immediately following diagnostic or interventional cardiac catheterization, successful deployment (hemostasis achieved within 2 minutes) was achieved in 92% of patients; 4% of patients developed a hematoma >10 cm and only 0.7% had a major complication. One case report describes the successful percutaneous closure of a patent foramen ovale using this device. No randomized controlled trials have yet been reported on this device.

X-Press (Datascope Corporation, Fairfield, NJ) is another percutaneous suture device that is fully nonmechanical consisting of a 6-Fr. over-the-wire catheter, a guidewire, a suture pack with a single strand of suture, two needles, and a knot pusher. Unlike Perclose or SuperStitch, the X-press device has no intraluminal moving parts, thereby limiting the risk of vessel dissection, ruptured plaque, or vessel occlusion. The RACE randomized controlled trial compared femoral artery closure with the X-Press device versus manual compression in patients who underwent diagnostic catheterization or PCI and demonstrated a significant reduction in time to ambulation in the X-Press arm. In the whole cohort of patients, rates of major complications were no different between the two treatment groups; however, **in the PCI patients, the rate of major complications was lower in the X-Press group** (0% in the X-press arm, 3.4% with manual compression, $p = 0.037$). Currently, this device can only be used for vascular sheaths up to 6 Fr. in size.

A trial comparing four different methods of arterial closure showed that the Perclose had a 2.3% incidence of major complications, inferior only to the Angio-Seal. Another large randomized trial found that the times to hemostasis, ambulation, and discharge were significantly lower in patients who received suture-mediated closure compared to manual pressure. The mean time to ambulation was 2 hours with suture-mediated closure and 6.5 hours with manual compression. However, a significantly higher incidence of vascular complications was noted in the suture-mediated closure group. Anticoagulated patients derived particular benefit from suture-mediated closure in regards to hemostasis, time to ambulation, and discharge.

Staple and Clip Devices: Staple and clip VCDs deliver a metallic extraluminal component that "cinches" the edges of the arteriotomy. The staples and clips are made of biologically inert metals (nitinol, titanium) thereby causing less of an inflammatory response than is often caused by the collagen-based biosealant devices.

The **StarClose** (Abbott Vascular, Abbott Labs, IL) VCD deploys a nitinol clip to the extraluminal side of the arterial wall that provides circumferential traction toward the arterial wall defect thereby closing the arteriotomy. A study comparing StarClose to Angio-Seal and manual compression found no significant difference in complication rate; however, patients in the StarClose arm were more likely to require additional compression after successful device deployment.

The **EVS Vascular Closure System** (angioLink Corporation, Taunton, MA) is a VCD that augments hemostasis by deploying an extraluminal titanium staple at the arteriotomy. It is composed of an introducer assembly with vessel dilator, a titanium staple, and a trigger-activated trigger deployment system (Figure 9-8). Advantages of this device include: (1) it can be used in large arteriotomies (>10 Fr.) and (2) **it can safely be used to close noncommon femoral arteriotomies (superficial and deep femoral arteries).** The device is utilized by removing the arterial sheath and advancing the dilator and introducer assembly into the lumen until there is blood return through a central lumen. The stabilization feet temporarily deployed in the lumen and retracted until gentle resistance is felt (the "feet" are against the vessel wall). The dilator is removed and the staple device is advanced through the introducer until gentle resistance is met

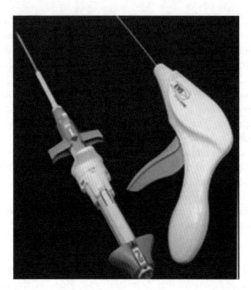

Figure **9-8** **EVS Vascular Closure System.** (From Caputo RP, Ebner A, Grant W, et al. Percutaneous femoral arteriotomy repair—initial experience with a novel staple closure device. *J Invasive Cardiol.* 2002;14:652–656.)

and then the staple is deployed. The stabilization feet are retracted and the introducer is removed. An uncontrolled prospective study of 89 consecutive arteriotomies closed by the EVS VCD reported 92% successful arterial closure and no complications.

Novel Devices: The **Catalyst Closure Device System** (Cardiva Medical Corporation, Sunnyvale, CA) is a new VCD that consists of an expandable nitinol mesh disk mounted on the end of an 18-gauge wire. The Catalyst II wire is inserted into the artery through the existing catheterization sheath (5 to 7 Fr.) and the nitinol disk is expanded in the vessel lumen. The nitinol disk is gently pulled against the artery wall as the sheath is removed and an external clip is applied to the wire, thereby maintaining site-specific hands-free compression of the arteriotomy and achieving hemostasis. The device is left in this position for an appropriate "dwell time" (15 minutes for a diagnostic case, 120 minutes after PCI) during which time the natural recoil of the vascular wall smooth muscle occurs, causing the arteriotomy size to decrease significantly. After the dwell time, the intraluminal disk is retracted, the wire is removed from the groin, and "fingertip" manual pressure is applied to the puncture site for 5 to 7 minutes. While no studies are yet available for the Catalyst II device, a prospective study of its precursor (the Boomerang Catalyst Device) reported a 99% rate of successful hemostasis with no major complications. Benefits of this device include no residual indwelling material and potentially minimal arterial wall and soft tissue scarring; a limitation is the need for some manual pressure.

The **Femoral Introducer Sheath and Hemostasis (FISH) device** (MIR Corporation, Bloomington, IN) is a novel product that combines access and closure on the same device. This unique device incorporates an extracellular matrix closure patch that is premounted onto a 5, 6, or 8 Fr. access sheath. A recent prospective randomized controlled trial of 297 patients demonstrated a significant reduction in time to hemostasis, time to ambulation, and time to discharge with the FISH device when compared to manual compression. There were higher rates of major or minor complications associated with use of the FISH device; however, these were not statistically significant. Ongoing research is needed to determine the safety and efficacy of this device compared with other methods of vascular closure.

Complications

Arterial puncture and cannulation is associated with significant vascular complications including hemorrhage, pseudoaneurysm, arteriovenous fistula, thrombosis, embolism, and infection; the occurrence of these is associated with increased morbidity and mortality (Table 9-1). The risk of vascular complications requiring surgery ranges from 0.5% to 1% following diagnostic catheterization, from 0.5% to 3% following balloon angioplasty, and up to 14% following coronary stenting. The clinical and procedure-related risk factors associated with vascular complications are listed in Table 9-2. In general, a higher rate of vascular occlusion (local thrombosis or distal embolization) occurs with the collagen-based

Table **9-1**	Vascular Complications
Potential Complications	
Pseudoaneurysm	
Arteriovenous fistula	
Hemorrhage	
Thrombosis	
Embolism	
Infection	

Table **9-2**	Risk Factors Associated with Increased Incidence of Vascular Complications

Risk Factors

Clinical Factors
Advanced age
Female gender
Smaller body surface area
Congestive heart failure
Peripheral vascular disease

Procedural Factors
Anticoagulation
Cardiac intervention (PTCA, atherectomy, valvuloplasty)
Use of larger sized sheaths

biosealant devices than with the percutaneous suture devices. Infection occurs more often with VCDs that deploy foreign material that is left at the arteriotomy site and severe perivascular infection and endarteritis have been described following the deployment of VCDs. As a result, many operators will resterilize the puncture site prior to utilization of a VCD.

Arterial Access Site and Sheath Size

6-Fr. catheter systems via the femoral artery remain the most widely used system for coronary angiography. However, smaller sheath size and radial artery access are increasingly being employed in an effort to reduce hospitalization time and complication rate. A substudy of the SYNERGY trial found a lower rate of hemorrhagic complications associated with radial artery access when compared to femoral artery access. Additionally, in the femoral artery arm, sheath size was directly proportional to rate of non-CABG TIMI-major bleeding (1.5% for 4 or 5 Fr., 1.6% for 6 Fr., 3.3% for 7 Fr., and 3.8% of 8 Fr., p <0.0001). Another trial comparing femoral artery access and closure with Angio-Seal or Starclose versus radial artery access found that radial artery access is associated with a lower rate of major complications and improved patient comfort; however, transradial access was also associated with longer procedural times and increased radiation exposure. Other studies report that the difference in procedural time and radiation exposure is overcome as operator experience with the transradial approach increases. A study comparing coronary angiography with 4-Fr. femoral artery access, 6-Fr.

femoral artery access with Angio-Seal closure, and radial artery access found similar times to ambulation and hospital discharge between the groups; however, use of a 4-Fr. system came at the cost of inferior angiographic image quality. Angiographic quality with a 4-Fr. system can be significantly improved when a contrast power injector is used.

Cost

Hospital length of stay and the need for trained personnel are major factors that contribute to the total cost of percutaneous cardiac procedures. One goal for VCDs is that their use will result in a shorter time to patient discharge and a decreased need for trained personnel and that these will directly translate into lower hospital costs. One study looking at the safety and cost associated with the use of Perclose versus manual compression in patients post PCI found no difference in complication rate, but did note a significant reduction in time to discharge and cost for patients in the Perclose arm. A similar study with the Duett device found a nonstatistically significant trend toward lower cost with the device versus manual compression. A cost-minimization analysis of use of the Angio-Seal device in patients post PCI predicted the use of Angio-Seal to be more cost-effective than manual pressure; however, a prospective study comparing the actual cost of Angio-Seal versus mechanical compression with the FemStop device found arterial closure with Angio-Seal to be more expensive. This was largely due to the difference in cost of the devices. A pilot study looking at the use of the Angio-Seal in patients who had undergone PCI found that same-day discharge was feasible and safe in select patients treated for stable angina. While this trial did not directly look at hospital cost, the authors noted that the dramatic reduction in time to hospital discharge would significantly reduce the cost of the procedure. Another study of patients undergoing diagnostic catheterization reported that use of a 6-Fr. system and Angio-Seal device closure was more costly than using a 4-Fr. system and manual pressure. Overall, these studies indicate that use of smaller catheters is likely more cost-effective and safe for diagnostic procedures. However, for patients undergoing PCI, the significant reduction in time to hospital discharge increasingly made possible by the use of VCDs will probably result in an ultimate reduction in cost as well.

Conclusions

Manual pressure has long been the gold standard for achieving hemostasis in patients after percutaneous cardiovascular procedures. However, many VCDs are now commercially available and they offer the advantages of early sheath removal, early ambulation, and early hospital discharge, as well as allow for uninterrupted anticoagulation when needed. As physicians have become more experienced with the newer generations of VCDs, the associated procedural complication rates associated with their use have been shown to be comparable or even lower than those associated with manual pressure. Smaller catheter sizes and radial artery access are being increasingly used for diagnostic coronary procedures and their use is associated with lower rates of complication and decreased costs when compared to VCDs. However, in interventional procedures, the significant reduction in time to hospital discharge and ability to not interrupt anticoagulation associated with VCDs make their use safe and likely more cost-effective.

Suggested Reading

Seldinger SI. Catheter replacement of the needle in percutaneous arteriography: a new technique. *Acta Radiol*. 1953;39:368–376.

Doyle BJ, Konz BA, Lennon RJ, et al. Ambulation 1 hour after diagnostic cardiac catheterization: a prospective study of 1009 procedures. *Mayo Clin Proc*. 2006;81:1537–1540.

Hallak OK, Cubeddu RJ, Griffith RA, et al. The use of the D-STAT dry bandage for the control of vascular access site bleeding: a multicenter experience in 376 patients. *Cardiovasc Intervent Radiol*. 2007;30:593–600.

D-Stat Dry Hemostatic Bandage Topical Hemostat. Minneapolis, MN: Vascular Solutions, Inc.; 2009.

Palmer BL, Gantt DS, Lawrence ME, et al. Effectiveness and safety of manual hemostasis facilitated by the SyvekPatch with one hour of bedrest after coronary angiography using six-French catheters. *Am J Cardiol*. 2004;93: 96–97.

Abbott WM, Austen WG. The effectiveness and mechanism of collagen-induced topical hemostasis. *Surgery*. 1975;78:723–729.

Blanc R, Mounayer C, Piotin M, et al. Hemostatic closure device after carotid puncture for stent and coil placement in an intracranial aneurysm: technical note. *AJNR Am J Neuroradiol*. 2002;23:978–981.

Massiere B, von Ristow A, Cury JM, et al. Closure of carotid artery puncture site with a percutaneous device. *Ann Vasc Surg*. 2009;23:256 e5–e7.

Micha JP, Goldstein BH, Lindsay SF, et al. Subclavian artery puncture repair with Angio-Seal deployment. *Gynecol Oncol*. 2007;104:761–763.

Petrov I, Dimitrov C. Closing of a right ventricle perforation with a vascular closure device. *Catheter Cardiovasc Interv*. 2009;74:247–250.

Mooney MR, Ellis SG, Gershony G, et al. Immediate sealing of arterial puncture sites after cardiac catheterization and coronary interventions: initial U.S. feasibility trial using the Duett vascular closure device. *Catheter Cardiovasc Interv*. 2000;50:96–102.

Michalis LK, Rees MR, Patsouras D, et al. A prospective randomized trial comparing the safety and efficacy of three commercially available closure devices (Angioseal, Vasoseal and Duett). *Cardiovasc Intervent Radiol*. 2002;25:423–429.

Shammas NW, Rajendran VR, Alldredge SG, et al. Randomized comparison of Vasoseal and Angioseal closure devices in patients undergoing coronary angiography and angioplasty. *Catheter Cardiovasc Interv.* 2002;55:421–425.

Bhatt DL, Raymond RE, Feldman T, et al. Successful "pre-closure" of 7 Fr and 8 Fr femoral arteriotomies with a 6 Fr suture-based device (the Multicenter Interventional Closer Registry). *Am J Cardiol.* 2002;89:777–779.

Hon LQ, Ganeshan A, Thomas SM, et al. Vascular closure devices: a comparative overview. *Curr Probl Diagn Radiol.* 2009;38:33–43.

Clinical Investigators Review Sutura Next Generation SuperStitch Vessel Closure Device. Business Wire.

Eggebrecht H, Naber C, Woertgen U, et al. Percutaneous suture-mediated closure of femoral access sites deployed through the procedure sheath: initial clinical experience with a novel vascular closure device. *Catheter Cardiovasc Interv.* 2003;58:313–321.

Ruiz CE, Kipshidze N, Chiam PT, et al. Feasibility of patent foramen ovale closure with no-device left behind: first-in-man percutaneous suture closure. *Catheter Cardiovasc Interv.* 2008;71:921–926.

Sanborn TA, Ogilby JD, Ritter JM, et al. Reduced vascular complications after percutaneous coronary interventions with a nonmechanical suture device: results from the randomized RACE study. *Catheter Cardiovasc Interv.* 2004; 61:327–332.

Ratnam LA, Raja J, Munneke GJ, et al. Prospective nonrandomized trial of manual compression and Angio-Seal and Starclose arterial closure devices in common femoral punctures. *Cardiovasc Intervent Radiol.* 2007;30:182–188.

Caputo RP, Ebner A, Grant W, et al. Percutaneous femoral arteriotomy repair—initial experience with a novel staple closure device. *J Invasive Cardiol.* 2002;14:652–656.

Cardiva Catalyst II Instructions for Use. Sunnyvale, CA: Cardiva Medical, Inc.; 2010.

Doyle BJ, Godfrey MJ, Lennon RJ, et al. Initial experience with the Cardiva Boomerang vascular closure device in diagnostic catheterization. *Catheter Cardiovasc Interv.* 2007;69:203–208.

Bavry AA, Raymond RE, Bhatt DL, et al. Efficacy of a novel procedure sheath and closure device during diagnostic catheterization: the multicenter randomized clinical trial of the FISH device. *J Invasive Cardiol.* 2008;20:152–156.

Bashore TM, Bates ER, Berger PB, et al. American College of Cardiology/Society for Cardiac Angiography and Interventions Clinical Expert Consensus Document on Cardiac Catheterization Laboratory Standards. A report of the American College of Cardiology Task Force on Clinical Expert Consensus Documents. *J Am Coll Cardiol.* 2001;37:2170–214.

Hoffer EK, Bloch RD. Percutaneous arterial closure devices. *J Vasc Interv Radiol.* 2003;14:865–885.

Lasic Z, Nikolsky E, Kesanakurthy S, et al. Vascular closure devices: a review of their use after invasive procedures. *Am J Cardiovasc Drugs.* 2005;5:185–200.

Cantor WJ, Mahaffey KW, Huang Z, et al. Bleeding complications in patients with acute coronary syndrome undergoing early invasive management can be reduced with radial access, smaller sheath sizes, and timely sheath removal. *Catheter Cardiovasc Interv.* 2007;69:73–83.

Sciahbasi A, Fischetti D, Picciolo A, et al. Transradial access compared with femoral puncture closure devices in percutaneous coronary procedures. *Int J Cardiol.* 2009;137:199–205.

Elgharib NZ, Shah UH, Coppola JT. Transradial cardiac catheterization and percutaneous coronary intervention: a review. *Coron Artery Dis.* 2009;20:487–493.

Reddy BK, Brewster PS, Walsh T, et al. Randomized comparison of rapid ambulation using radial, 4 French femoral access, or femoral access with AngioSeal closure. *Catheter Cardiovasc Interv.* 2004;62:143–149.

Rickli H, Unterweger M, Sutsch G, et al. Comparison of costs and safety of a suture-mediated closure device with conventional manual compression after coronary artery interventions. *Catheter Cardiovasc Interv.* 2002;57:297–302.

Zhang Z, Mahoney EM, Gershony G, et al. Impact of the Duett sealing device on quality of life and hospitalization costs for coronary diagnostic and interventional procedures: results from the Study of Economic and Quality of Life substudy of the SEAL trial. *Am Heart J.* 2001;142:982–988.

Resnic FS, Arora N, Matheny M, et al. A cost-minimization analysis of the angioseal vascular closure device following percutaneous coronary intervention. *Am J Cardiol.* 2007;99:766–770.

Juergens CP, Leung DY, Crozier JA, et al. Patient tolerance and resource utilization associated with an arterial closure versus an external compression device after percutaneous coronary intervention. *Catheter Cardiovasc Interv.* 2004;63:166–170.

Yee KM, Lazzam C, Richards J, et al. Same-day discharge after coronary stenting: a feasibility study using a hemostatic femoral puncture closure device. *J Interv Cardiol.* 2004;17:315–320.

CHAPTER 10

Post-Cath Complications

*Arun Kalyanasundaram
and Mehdi H. Shishehbor*

Although a relatively safe procedure, cardiac catheterization carries a low but significant risk of both major and minor complications. The combined complication of contrast media reaction, cardiogenic shock, cerebrovascular accident, congestive heart failure, cardiac tamponade, and renal failure following a diagnostic catheterization is <2%, and the risk of mortality is 0.1% (0.6 in a 1,000).

A brief history should be elicited to detect any symptoms suggestive of potential complications (Table 10-1).

The post-catheterization examination accordingly needs to focus on likely complications and should be directed by the history. The vital signs should be reviewed and blood pressure and pulse checked in supine and erect position if possible. The presence of tachycardia after cardiac catheterization should always prompt a search for the underlying cause. It may be a manifestation of intravascular depletion secondary to diuresis or bleeding or a sign of decompensated heart failure. It may also be a marker of pericardial irritation. Fever immediately after catheterization is not normal and may be a pyrogen reaction to fluids or medications. Any fever should prompt a search for an infective focus.

A brief neurologic examination should routinely be performed, and special attention should be paid to the patient's speech and gait. Importantly, patients may not note neurologic deficits until they ambulate; these may include focal paresis or paralysis, visual symptoms, sensory deficits, and ataxia.

The jugular venous pressure should be assessed as an index of intravascular status, while cardiac auscultation should focus on the presence of any pericardial rub. All patients who have had subclavian or jugular cannulation need to be examined for signs of pneumothorax, as it may not manifest during the procedure.

Table **10-1**	Symptoms Suggestive of Cardiac Catheterization Complications
Symptom	**Differential Diagnoses**
Chest pain	Coronary ischemia
	Aortic dissection
	Coronary perforation
	Cardiac perforation
Dyspnea	Coronary ischemia
	Congestive heart failure
	Pneumothorax
Groin pain	Localized bleeding
Leg pain/numbness	Femoral nerve compression
	Femoral artery dissection
	Femoral artery thrombosis
	Local nerve block from anesthetic
Flank pain	Retroperitoneal bleed
Nausea/hiccups	Hemopericardium

Local Complications

The most important part of the examination that is unique to the post-cath check is the assessment of the catheterization site. The site of catheterization should be checked for evidence of bleeding, pseudoaneurysm, arteriovenous fistula (a new onset bruit), or vascular compromise (absent distal pulses). Factors associated with high risk of local bleeding include advanced age, female gender, low body mass index (BMI), and use of anticoagulants or platelet glycoprotein IIb/IIIa inhibitors. **Fluoroscopy prior to obtaining access routinely has been shown to reduce the complication rate significantly**. Bleeding has been recognized increasingly as an important predictor of increased mortality. Due to their associated morbidity and mortality, we will discuss post-catheterization bleeding, pseudoaneurysm, and infection in greater detail.

Hematoma: Bleeding after cardiac catheterization may be external or may manifest as a hematoma. Clinically, hematomas present as pain or local discomfort, focal discoloration or bruising, hemodynamic compromise, and rarely as femoral nerve compression and quadriceps weakness.

Meticulous detail to puncture technique by using external and internal landmarks and avoidance of multiple or posterior wall puncture will reduce the incidence of local bleeding. When using fluoroscopy, attention should be given to the presence of calcium. In general, the femoral puncture should be above or below any calcification if possible. Other measures to reduce the frequency and severity of groin bleeding include careful monitoring of anticoagulation and careful attention to hemostasis during sheath removal. Adequate hemostasis must be achieved with manual pressure or a closure device before leaving the patient's bedside (Figure 10-1).

Retroperitoneal Hematoma: Retroperitoneal hematoma is usually associated with arterial puncture above the inguinal ligament. Hence, routine angiography of the common femoral artery might be reasonable even in diagnostic procedures to determine the risk of this complication. Since all the bleeding may be internal, the patient often presents with unexplained hypotension and tachycardia (occasionally bradycardia) without any external signs. Flank pain and bruising may be seen in some patients. An unexplained falling hematocrit may be the only finding in others. Dysuria might also be a presenting symptom as the hematoma presses on the bladder.

The best modality for detection of a retroperitoneal hematoma is a computed tomography (CT) scan. Ultrasound may be used if CT is not available. Since the therapy of retroperitoneal hematoma is based on its clinical implications, and directed toward correcting those, some physicians do not routinely obtain radiologic imaging studies. Unstable patients should not be sent for a CT scan. A conservative strategy of reserving these tests for patients where a definitive diagnosis is required to guide therapy, such as determining the need for withholding anticoagulant or antiplatelet therapy in stable patients might be reasonable.

Pseudoaneurysm: Pseudoaneurysm is defined as arterial wall disruption with resultant extraluminal flow into a chamber contained by adjacent tissue. Arterial tissue does not contribute to the wall of the pseudoaneurysm. The incidence of pseudoaneurysm has varied between

Troubleshooting

Management of retroperitoneal hematoma: The mainstay of therapy for a hematoma or retroperitoneal hematoma consists of volume resuscitation and blood transfusion if appropriate. Further anticoagulants and platelet antagonists should be withheld. The decision to reverse anticoagulation and transfuse platelets in patients receiving platelet glycoprotein IIb/IIIa inhibitors or platelet adenosine diphosphate (ADP) antagonists (ticlopidine or clopidogrel) should be individualized for each patient. Patients could be taken back to the cardiac catheterization suite, and the vascular system imaged via contralateral access. Endovascular intervention is a definite option, especially if identified early in the course of the development of the hematoma.

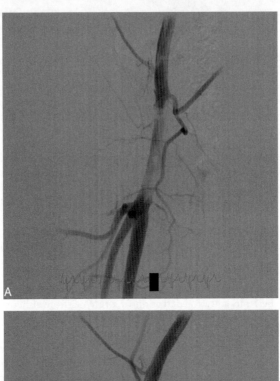

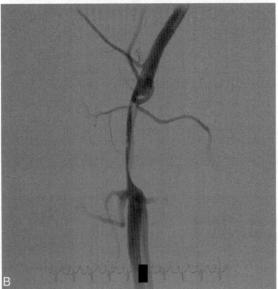

Figure **10-1** **A)** Dissection of the common femoral artery extending from the distal external iliac into and involving the entire common femoral artery with extensive compromise of the true lumen with an 80% stenosis from compression by the false lumen, which is full of thrombus. **B)** On the right anterior oblique angiogram, the footplate and collagen plug from the Angio-Seal device are visualized.

0.3% and 0.5% of cardiac catheterizations in large series. In a recent study of patients treated with platelet glycoprotein IIb/IIIa inhibitors, pseudoaneurysms were noted in 0.5% of patients treated with manual pressure, 0.8% of patients treated with Angio-Seal, and 0.4% of patients treated with Perclose.

A pseudoaneurysm may present with pain, new bruit, and pulsatile mass, expanding hematoma, or leg weakness. The best diagnostic imaging modality for a pseudoaneurysm is a color flow duplex ultrasonography. The pseudoaneurysm is occasionally multichambered. The mean transverse diameter of pseudoaneurysms in a recently published series was 2.46 cm by 2.14 cm. The majority of the pseudoaneurysms in this study arose from the common femoral artery with the average pseudoaneurysm tract length of 1.4 cm, and the average depth of the pseudoaneurysm neck arising from the native artery of 30.2 mm (Figure 10-2).

A pseudoaneurysm may rupture or lead to thromboembolism, neurovascular compression, or pressure necrosis. The risk factors for pseudoaneurysm have included multiple arterial punctures, superficial femoral artery puncture, large sheath size, arterial hypertension, and antiplatelet or antithrombotic therapy. Of note, pseudoaneurysms that

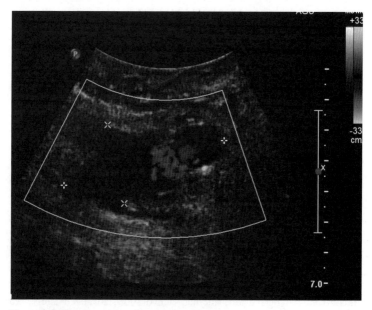

Figure **10-2**   Femoral artery pseudoaneurysm.

Troubleshooting

Management of femoral artery pseudoaneurysm: Ultrasound-guided thrombin injection (UGTI) is the preferred method of treatment in most cases with a success rate >90%. Ultrasound-guided compression was the most commonly used therapy prior to the advent of UGTI, but it was associated with a failure rate 5% to 15%. Surgical repair has been associated with a high risk of complications predominantly due to the associated comorbidities in this group of patients. There have been small case series of successful use of endovascular-covered stents to treat pseudoaneurysms.

are less than 2 cm are of no major consequence and should only be monitored.

Infections: Groin infection is a rare complication of cardiac catheterization. This is rarely seen with manual compression (reported incidence, 0–0.05%), but its incidence is higher in patients receiving closure devices (0–0.3%). The most commonly implicated organism is *Staphylococcus aureus*. Patients often present with groin pain, groin erythema, purulent discharge, fever, and leucocytosis. Since cardiac catheterization is inherently a sterile procedure, infection is usually secondary to breakdown in sterile technique. Careful attention must be paid to the condition of skin at the access site prior to insertion of the sheath, and an alternate site should be selected if there are concerns about dermal integrity. While some physicians administer periprocedural antibiotics to patients receiving closure devices, there is no randomized controlled data to support such a practice. The lack of proven benefit must be weighed against the risk of drug allergy, superinfection, drug resistance, and cost.

The therapy for groin infection includes appropriate antibiotics and surgical debridement if indicated. Early consultation with a vascular surgeon is advisable.

Contrast-induced Nephropathy (CIN): CIN is a complication defined as new onset or exacerbation of renal dysfunction after contrast administration. The risk is directly related to baseline renal function. CIN is defined as either a relative increase in serum creatinine of ≥25% above the baseline value, or an absolute increase >0.5 mg/dL of creatinine, and it typically develops about 24 to 48 hours post contrast exposure. Risk factors for development of CIN include baseline renal insufficiency, diabetes mellitus, left ventricular ejection fraction (LVEF) <40%, uncontrolled hypertension, anemia, dehydration, advanced age (>75 years), use of diuretics, other nephrotoxic medications, and volume of contrast used. **Adequate hydration pre- and post-catheterization is the best strategy to reduce the incidence of CIN.** Initial studies suggested that hydration with sodium bicarbonate before contrast exposure was more effective than hydration with sodium chloride for prophylaxis of contrast-induced renal failure, although a systematic review concluded that the effectiveness remains uncertain. N-acetylcysteine likely reduces the incidence of contrast nephropathy, although this has not been consistently demonstrated. Given the virtual lack of side effects and possible benefit, utilization is recommended in patients with impaired glomerular filtration rate (GFR). Most episodes of CIN resolve over time with careful hydration and monitoring. In addition to CIN, atheroembolic-associated renal insufficiency should also be considered. In general, urine eosinophils are checked. However, the management of this condition is similar to CIN and requires hydration and time.

Physical Limitations Post-Catheterization

All patients are advised to restrict activities for a short duration of time to permit adequate healing of the access site. Table 10-2 outlines commonly prescribed minimum restrictions for patients after cardiac catheterization at a major medical center. Some patients may be advised

Table **10-2**	Activity Restriction Following Cardiac Catheterization
Approach	**Activity Restriction**
Brachial	Dressing to be removed after 1 day
	Keep site clean and dry
	No strenuous activity **until sutures removed** (cutdown)
	or **48 hours** (Seldinger technique)
	Not to lift >10 lb
	No bowling or tennis
	No activity that involves excessive pushing or pulling with involved arm
Femoral	Can resume normal activity after 24 hours
	No swimming or bath (can shower) for a week if closure device used
	For the first 24 hours
	No driving
	No lifting of objects >10 lb
	No climbing, cycling, or any other strenuous activity

to restrict their activities further on the basis of the findings of their cardiac catheterization.

Indications for Routine Labs

No labs need to be checked routinely after diagnostic cardiac catheterization. In patients suspected of bleeding, the hematocrit should be checked as necessary. Renal function is checked after 48 hours in patients with known renal insufficiency who are suspected to be at risk for CIN. In our program we routinely assess cardiac enzymes post procedure, however, this is not mandatory unless indicated clinically.

Suggested Reading

Aguirre FV, Topol EJ, Ferguson JJ, et al. Bleeding complications with the chimeric antibody to platelet glycoprotein IIb/IIIa integrin in patients undergoing percutaneous coronary intervention. EPIC Investigators. *Circulation.* 1995;91:2882–2890.

Amini M, Salarifar M, Amirbaigloo A, et al. N-acetylcysteine does not prevent contrast-induced nephropathy after cardiac catheterization in patients with diabetes mellitus and chronic kidney disease: a randomized clinical trial. *Trials.* 2009;10:45.

Applegate RJ, Little WC, Craven T, et al. Vascular closure devices in patients treated with anticoagulation and IIb/IIIa receptor inhibitors during percutaneous revascularization. *J Am Coll Cardiol.* 2002;40:78–83.

Cherr GS, Travis JA, Ligush J Jr, et al. Infection is an unusual but serious complication of a femoral artery catheterization site closure device. *Ann Vasc Surg.* 2001;15:567–570.

Cooper CL, Miller A. Infectious complications related to the use of the Angio-seal hemostatic puncture closure device. *Catheter Cardiovasc Interv.* 1999;48:301–303.

Davidson CJ, Hlatky M, Morris KG, et al. Cardiovascular and renal toxicity of a nonionic radiographic contrast agent after cardiac catheterization. A prospective trial. *Ann Intern Med.* 1989;110(2):119–124.

Doyle BJ, Rihal CS, Gastineau DA, et al. Bleeding, blood transfusion, and increased mortality after percutaneous coronary intervention: implications for contemporary practice. *J Am Coll Cardiol.* 2009;53(22):2019–2127.

Fitts J, Ver Lee P, Hofmaster P, et al. Fluoroscopy-guided femoral artery puncture reduces the risk of PCI-related vascular complications. *J Interv Cardiol.* 2008;21(3):273–278.

La Perna L, Olin JW, Goines D, et al. Ultrasound-guided thrombin injection for the treatment of postcatheterization pseudoaneurysms. *Circulation.* 2000;102:2391–2395.

Lumsden AB, Miller JM, Kosinski AS, et al. A prospective evaluation of surgically treated groin complications following percutaneous cardiac procedures. *Am Surg.* 1994;60:132–137.

Merten GJ, Burgess WP, Gray LV, et al. Prevention of contrast-induced nephropathy with sodium bicarbonate: a randomized controlled trial. *JAMA.* 2004;291(19):2328–2334.

Rosamond W, Flegal K, Friday G, et al. Heart disease and stroke statistics—2007 update: a report from the American Heart Association Statistics Committee and Stroke Statistics Subcommittee. *Circulation.* 2007;115(5):e69–e171.

Rudnick MR, Goldfarb S, Wexler L, et al. Nephrotoxicity of ionic and nonionic contrast media in 1196 patients: a randomized trial. The Iohexol Cooperative Study. *Kidney Int.* 1995;47(1):254–261.

Sohail MR, Khan AH, Holmes DR Jr, et al. Infectious complications of percutaneous vascular closure devices. *Mayo Clin Proc.* 2005;80(8):1011–1015.

Thalhammer C, Kirchherr AS, Uhlich F, et al. Postcatheterization pseudoaneurysms and arteriovenous fistulas: repair with percutaneous implantation of endovascular covered stents. *Radiology.* 2000;214:127–131.

Trivedi H, Daram S, Szabo A, et al. High-dose *N*-acetylcysteine for the prevention of contrast-induced nephropathy. *Am J Med.* 2009;122(9):874 e9–874 e15.

Waigand J, Uhlich F, Gross CM, et al. Percutaneous treatment of pseudoaneurysms and arteriovenous fistulas after invasive vascular procedures. *Catheter Cardiovasc Interv.* 1999;47:157–164.

Zoungas S, Ninomiya T, Huxley R, et al. Systematic review: sodium bicarbonate treatment regimens for the prevention of contrast-induced nephropathy. *Ann Intern Med.* 2009;151(9):631–638.

CHAPTER 11

Study Questions

1. Absolute contraindications to cardiac catheterization include:
   a. Acute renal failure
   b. Decompensated congestive heart failure
   c. Severe hypokalemia
   d. Patient's refusal to undergo cardiac catheterization
   e. All of the above

2. Medications that should be withheld prior to cardiac catheterization include:
   a. Aspirin
   b. Metformin
   c. Unfractionated heparin
   d. Clopidogrel
   e. None of the above

3. True or false. Renal atheroembolic disease accounts for the majority of acute renal failure cases following cardiac catheterization procedures.

4. True or false. Contrast reactions are allergic reactions mediated by immunoglobulin E (IgE).

5. The main source of radiation exposure to the operator is from:
   a. Escape of x-rays through the shielding of the x-ray tube
   b. Forgetting to wear lead during the cardiac catheterization
   c. Scatter from the patient
   d. All of the above contribute equally to operator radiation exposure

6. Techniques used to minimize radiation exposure include which of the following:
   a. Personal lead shielding
   b. Taking a step back from the irradiated area before engaging in fluoroscopy
   c. Keeping beam-on time to an absolute minimum
   d. All of the above

7. Coronary artery "dominance" is determined by:
   a. Size of the coronary artery; right-dominant in approximately 85% of cases
   b. Artery that gives rise to the posterior descending artery; left-dominant in approximately 15% of cases

179

   c. Artery that gives rise to the posterior descending artery; codominant in approximately 15% of cases

   d. Artery that gives rise to the atrioventricular (AV) node artery; right-dominant in approximately 85% of cases

   e. Artery that gives rise to the posterior descending artery; right-dominant in approximately 85% of cases

8. A "ventricularized" waveform results from:
   a. A deep-seated catheter, restricting coronary inflow
   b. A catheter within the left ventricular cavity
   c. Significant left main coronary artery stenosis
   d. Both a and b
   e. Both a and c

9. To minimize the risk of coronary dissection when using the Amplatz catheters, the operator should:
   a. Rotate the catheter counterclockwise to disengage it from the coronary ostium prior to removing the catheter
   b. Withdraw the catheter straight back to disengage the coronary ostium
   c. Rotate the catheter clockwise to disengage it from the coronary ostium prior to removing the catheter
   d. Not use this catheter

10. The most common coronary anomaly is:
   a. Origin of the left main trunk from the right sinus of Valsalva
   b. Origin of the right coronary artery from the left sinus of Valsalva
   c. Origin of the left circumflex coronary artery from the right sinus of Valsalva
   d. Left anterior descending and left circumflex arteries arising from separate ostia
   e. Both a and c
   f. Both b and c
   g. Both c and d

11. Since the Gorlin equation for calculation of aortic valve area is somewhat complicated, the simplified Hakki formula is frequently used preferentially. In which circumstance(s) might the formula be inaccurate?
   a. Low transvalvular gradient
   b. Severe aortic stenosis (valve area <0.8 cm^2)
   c. High cardiac output
   d. Sinus tachycardia (>100 bpm)
   e. a and d

12. Which of the following is considered the gold standard (most accurate) for cardiac output measurement?
   a. Pulmonary artery thermodilution
   b. Fick technique

   c. Quantitative ventriculography
   d. All of the above are equally accurate

13. What is normal mixed venous oxygen saturation (Svo$_2$)?
   a. 35%
   b. 50%
   c. 60%
   d. 75%

14. Relative contraindications for ventriculography include:
   a. Elevated left ventricular end diastolic pressure
   b. Severe fibrocalcific aortic stenosis
   c. Severe left main stenosis
   d. Reduced creatinine clearance
   e. All of the above

15. When inserting a Swan-Ganz (pulmonary artery) catheter, the balloon should be inflated in the:
   a. Femoral vein
   b. Right atrium
   c. Right ventricle
   d. Pulmonary artery

16. Which radiographic projection for aortography is preferred to identify type A aortic dissection?
   a. Left anterior oblique projection
   b. Right anterior oblique projection
   c. Steep antero-posterior (AP) cranial projection
   d. Shallow AP caudal projection

17. Aneurysmal left ventricular wall motion bulges outward in systole. This movement is termed:
   a. Akinesis
   b. Dyskinesis
   c. Hypokinesis
   d. Asyneresis

18. Aorto-coronary bypass grafts anastomosed to the left coronary system may be cannulated with any of the following except:
   a. Amplatz left 2 (AL2)
   b. Multipurpose A (MPA)
   c. Judkins left 4 (JL4)
   d. Left coronary bypass (LCB)
   e. Judkins right 4 (JR4)

19. The best diagnostic catheter for an aorto-coronary bypass graft to the right coronary artery (RCA) with a steep inferior angulation at the ostium is:
    a. Multipurpose B (MPB)
    b. JR4
    c. Short-tip Judkins right
    d. Right coronary bypass (RCB)
    e. Hockey stick

20. From the distal to proximal (closest to aortic valve) ascending aorta, the order of coronary bypass grafts is:
    a. Left anterior descending (LAD), diagonal, left circumflex (LCX)
    b. Left circumflex, diagonal, LAD
    c. Diagnosed, the circumflex, LAD
    d. LAD, left circumflex, diagonal

21. The best view to assess the left internal mammary artery (LIMA) to LAD anastomosis is:
    a. Straight postero-anterior (PA) cranial
    b. Left anterior oblique (LAO) 50°, caudal 30°
    c. Straight PA caudal
    d. 90° lateral

22. What is the best view when performing ascending aortography to identify potential grafts to LAD or LCX?
    a. Straight PA cranial
    b. Straight PA caudal
    c. Right anterior oblique (RAO) 35° to 40°
    d. LAO 35° to 40°

23. When having difficulty cannulating upward takeoff bypass grafts with JR or Coronary Bypass Graft (LCB or RCB) catheters, the next best catheter to use is:
    a. Multipurpose B1
    b. Multipurpose A1
    c. Amplatz right 2 (AR2)
    d. Amplatz left 2 (AL2)

24. The best technique to prevent postcatheterization groin complication is:
    a. Use of fluoroscopy and bony landmarks
    b. Use of ultrasound and micropuncture needle
    c. Use of minimal local sedation
    d. Radial approach

25. The best way to minimize contrast-induced nephropathy (CIN) is:
    a. *N*-acetylcysteine 600 mg by mouth twice daily for 4 doses
    b. Sodium bicarbonate infusion

c. Low-osmolar nonionic contrast
d. Using the least amount of contrast as possible
e. All of the above

26. The best closure device for a calcified and diseased common femoral artery is:
    a. Manual compression
    b. FemStop
    c. Perclose
    d. Angio-Seal

27. The only vascular closure device that allows re-entry with a 0.035 wire after sheath has been removed is:
    a. Angio-Seal
    b. Perclose
    c. Starclose
    d. Mynx

28. The best method to treat common femoral artery pseudoaneurysm is:
    a. Covered stent
    b. Surgical correction
    c. Ultrasound-guided compression
    d. Ultrasound-guided thrombin injection

29. What is the best management approach for a common femoral and external iliac artery dissection when placing a femoral sheath?
    a. Surgical consultation
    b. Obtaining access in the opposite groin and evaluating the dissection from the contralateral side
    c. Placing a self-expanding stent via the ipsilateral groin
    d. Performing balloon angioplasty followed by covered stent placement

30. Complications from closure devices include:
    a. Retroperitoneal bleed
    b. Pseudoaneurysm formation
    c. Intermittent claudication
    d. All of the above

31. True or false. Closure devices are absolutely contraindicated when using a 4-Fr. or 5-Fr. sheath.

Case 1 (Questions 32 and 33)
A 69-year-old diabetic man with a history of bypass surgery 10 years ago and severe peripheral vascular disease presents to the emergency department complaining 4 hours of substernal chest pain, nausea, vomiting, and shortness of breath.

On exam, he is diaphoretic, his blood pressure is 90/68 mm Hg, and his pulse oximetry is 91%. Lung exam reveals bibasilar rales and his EKG shows diffuse ST segment depression. Bedside troponin is positive. He is taken emergently to the cath lab. Arterial access is difficult. The patient's condition continues to deteriorate. His blood pressure is 80/62 mm Hg, heart rate is 115 beats per minute (sinus tachycardia), and his respiratory rate is 30 breaths per minute. He is sedated and intubated. His blood pressure after endotracheal intubation is 65/48 mm Hg, heart rate is 95 beats per minute, and pulse oximetry is 70%. FiO_2 on the ventilator is 100%.

32. Hypotension in this patient is best explained by which of the following?
    a. Cardiogenic shock
    b. Acute retroperitoneal bleed
    c. Endotracheal intubation
    d. Vagal reaction
    e. a and c

33. Sudden hypoxemia in this patient is best explained by:
    a. Pulmonary edema
    b. Anaphylactic reaction to lidocaine
    c. Barotrauma (i.e., pneumothorax)
    d. Right-to-left intrapulmonary shunt

34. The best view for selective renal arteriography is:
    a. Straight AP projection
    b. Shallow left anterior oblique projection
    c. Shallow right anterior oblique projection
    d. Steep left anterior oblique projection

Case 2 (Questions 35 and 36)
A 72-year-old man with history of peripheral vascular disease and diabetes presents with a 1-week history of progressively worsening exertional chest pressure. The past 12 hours he has experienced two 15-minute episodes of resting chest discomfort associated to diaphoresis. He is evaluated in the emergency department after his second episode. In the emergency department, he is pain free and his EKG shows new deep T wave inversions in the anterior precordial leads. Four months prior to presentation, he underwent percutaneous revascularization with stenting of left external iliac artery and femoropopliteal bypass on the right. On exam, an Allen test on the right is positive (i.e., insufficient ulnar collateral flow). He has a normal femoral pulse on the right and 1+ femoral pulse on the left. He is taken to the cath lab urgently for cardiac catheterization and possible coronary revascularization.

35. True or false. It is safe to access the femoropoliteal bypass graft on the right.

36. The left femoral approach is selected. If difficulty is encountered obtaining access, the following techniques should be used except:
    a. Doppler needle guidance
    b. Micropuncture needle kit
    c. Continue repeated attempts using routine access needle
    d. Fluoroscopic guidance

37. The best view to visualize the iliac arteries includes:
    a. Contralateral angulation
    b. Ipsilateral angulation
    c. Straight PA

Answers

1. **d.** The only absolute contraindication to cardiac catheterization is a patient's refusal to undergo the procedure. Acute renal failure, decompensated congestive heart failure, and severe hypokalemia are all relative contraindications. The risks and potential benefits for cardiac catheterization should be assessed prior to pursuing the procedure in these circumstances. Additional scenarios that pose an increased risk of cardiac catheterization include active bleeding, acute stroke, malignant hypertension, untreated active infection, digitalis toxicity, aortic valve endocarditis, severe anemia or coagulopathy, and reduced life expectancy.

2. **b.** Metformin should be held the day prior to the procedure and restarted 2 days after the procedure if renal function remains unchanged. Metformin is eliminated primarily via the kidneys and therefore accumulates among patients with renal insufficiency (glomerular filtration rate <70 mL/min, or serum creatinine >1.6 mg/dL). Contrast media can impair renal function and lead to further retention of metformin, which is known to precipitate the onset of lactic acidosis. The incidence of lactic acidosis associated with metformin, regardless of exposure to contrast media, is 0.03 cases per 1,000 patients per year, and 50% result in death. There is no conclusive evidence to indicate that contrast media precipitates the development of metformin-induced lactic acidosis among patients with normal serum creatinine (<1.5 mg/dL). This complication is almost exclusively observed among non–insulin dependent diabetic patients with abnormal renal function before injection of contrast media.

   In patients who are candidates for percutaneous coronary intervention after diagnostic angiography, aspirin 325 mg should be administered on the day of the procedure. The use of clopidogrel (600 mg loading dose) prior to catheterization may be indicated in patients who are likely to undergo percutaneous coronary intervention. This must be weighed against the possibility that they will require coronary artery bypass graft surgery, which often must be postponed for several days after administration of clopidogrel. Warfarin should be stopped several days before the procedure. Ideally, the international normalized ratio should be less than 1.5 to 1.8 prior to catheterization, depending on operator comfort and acuity of the indication. Heparin (3,000 to 5,000 units IV) should be considered for patients undergoing cardiac catheterization via an arm approach. It is also reasonable to pursue cardiac catheterization in patients on unfractionated heparin; however, great care must be taken to achieve an anterior artery wall arteriotomy in order to minimize the risk of bleeding.

3. **False.** Renal dysfunction can result from administration of contrast agents, which is reported to occur in approximately 5% patients, or from renal atheroembolic disease, which is significantly less common. Renal atheroembolic disease complicates approximately 0.15% of cardiac catheterizations and should be suspected when acute renal failure occurs in conjunction with other clinical signs of embolization such as discolored toes, livedo reticularis, systemic or urinary eosinophilia, and abdominal pain.

4. **False.** A great deal of controversy exists regarding the exact mechanism of contrast reactions, but it is thought that the majority of reactions are not mediated by immunoglobin E, and thus are not truly allergic. Multiple investigators have demonstrated conclusively, however, that immediate reactions involve the granular release of histamine by mast cells and basophils, producing an anaphylactoid response. Regardless of the mechanism, the risk of a reaction to contrast is increased twofold in patients with a strong history of allergy or atopy such as asthma. A common misconception is that a prior reaction to seafood confers a greatly elevated risk of an adverse reaction with contrast exposure. In reality, patients with allergies to seafood have a similar risk of contrast reactions as those who have a strong history of other allergic reactions. Patients with a previous adverse reaction to contrast have about a sixfold increased risk of an adverse reaction upon repeat exposure to contrast when compared with individuals without a prior adverse reaction. This elevated risk justifies pharmacologic prophylaxis with steroids and histamine blockade prior to planned repeat contrast exposure for patients with a history of moderate or severe reactions, although it should be noted that data is very limited on the efficacy of these preventive pharmacologic measures when modern-day nonionic low osmolar contrast media (LOCM) or iso-osmolar contrast media (IOCM) is used. Physicians should also note that serious life-threatening reactions have been reported despite the use of steroid and antihistamine prophylaxis.

5. **c.** The main source of radiation exposure for the operator is scatter from the patient. A secondary, less significant, source is escape of x-rays through the shielding of the x-ray tube. Protection for the operator consists of shielding, proper positioning from the radiation source, and adjusting the fluoroscopic controls in an attempt to minimize radiation exposure while maintaining a high-quality image.

6. **d.** Personal shielding involves lead aprons, thyroid collars, and lead glasses. Lead aprons should have shielding properties equivalent to 0.5 mm of lead, which shields the covered areas of the operator from roughly 90% of scatter radiation. Lead glasses protect the operator from possible radiation-induced cataracts and should have side shields to decrease radiation from the lateral direction. Thyroid shields prevent large cumulative doses of radiation that could lead to thyroid cancer. These items should be checked annually with fluoroscopy to inspect for possible cracks, holes, and other signs of deterioration. The catheterization table will commonly have two lead shields: one which is a table side drape that protects the lower body of the operator, and one which is an adjustable lead acrylic shield that is suspended from the ceiling to aid in the protection of the operator's head and upper torso.

   The inverse square law addresses the important concept that radiation dose drops rapidly by the inverse square of the relative increase of distance from the radiation source. Operators can decrease their radiation exposure by taking a step back from the irradiated area before engaging in fluoroscopy. Moving the image intensifier, which is located above the patient, to as close to the patient as possible also reduces scatter radiation by reducing geometric magnification (radiation dose usually increases with the square of the magnification). Placing hands in the direct beam of radiation should only be done in cases of emergency.

Modifying fluoroscopic controls can also decrease radiation exposure for both the operator and the patient; however, these modifications may occasionally reduce image quality. One of the "golden rules" for minimizing radiation exposure is keeping beam-on time to an absolute minimum. Fluoroscopy or cineangiography should not be engaged if the image on the monitor is not being used. Most fluoroscopic machines have an option that allows the operator to select the level of image quality (low, normal, high). Low image quality reduces radiation dose rate, but often produces a noisy image. These images may be acceptable in certain situations such as checking position of a guidewire or catheter. Most fluoroscopic machines have pulsed fluoroscopy which results in x-rays being produced in short bursts instead of a continuous stream as in conventional fluoroscopy. Reducing the pulse frequency to 15 or 7.5 pulses of x-rays/second will reduce radiation exposure at the cost of producing a somewhat flickering, choppy image. A similar result is seen when one reduces the cine frame rate. Applying collimators (blades outside the x-ray tube that block x-rays) to the area of interest not only reduces scatter radiation to the operator but also improves image quality.

7. **e.** The posterior descending artery, which courses in the posterior interventricular groove, determines coronary dominance. In 85% of the cases, the posterior descending artery arises from the right coronary artery, making the coronary circulation right-dominant. In 7% of the cases, the circulation is codominant, with the posterior interventricular groove being supplied by both the right coronary artery and the left circumflex coronary artery. In 8% of the cases, the posterior descending artery arises from the left circumflex, making it the dominant artery.

8. **e.** A dampened pressure waveform (drop in the catheter tip systolic pressure) or a ventricularized pressure waveform (drop in the catheter tip diastolic pressure) usually indicates that the catheter tip is either deep-seated, restricting coronary inflow, or the tip is against the wall. It also indicates the possibility of significant left main stenosis. *This can be a dangerous situation that needs to be recognized quickly.* The catheter tip should be immediately withdrawn from the ostium. The ostium can be re-engaged cautiously. If a small injection of dye reveals significant ostial left main stenosis (another clue may be the absence of dye reflux into the aortic root with the injection), two short cine runs aimed at visualizing distal targets for bypass surgery should promptly be performed, and the catheter then immediately pulled back from the ostium. Care must be taken to avoid multiple engagements of the left main trunk as this can lead to abrupt vessel closure. In cases where significant left main trunk stenosis is suspected, the operator can take nonselective angiograms of the left main trunk by injecting dye with the catheter tip positioned in left sinus. Catheter damping may also be seen in cases of spasm of the left main trunk.

In such instances, intracoronary nitroglycerin can be injected (200 μg) and follow-up picture can be taken to document relief of spasm.

9. **a.** To minimize the risk of coronary dissection when using the Amplatz catheters, the operator should rotate the catheter counterclockwise to disengage it from the coronary ostium prior to removing the catheter. Withdrawing the Amplatz catheters straight back will cause the catheter to "dive" into the coronary artery and increase the risk of dissection.

10. **g.** The various coronary anomalies in order of frequency are as follows: left anterior descending and left circumflex arteries arising from separate ostia (0.5%); origin of the left circumflex coronary artery from the right sinus of Valsalva (0.5%); origin of the right coronary artery from the ascending aorta above the right sinus of Valsalva (0.2%); origin of the right coronary artery from the left sinus of Valsalva (0.1%); AV fistula (0.1%); origin of the left main trunk from the right sinus of Valsalva (0.02%).

11. **d.** The Hakki formula calculates valve area (in cm^2) by dividing the cardiac output (in L/min) by the square root of the peak pressure gradient across the valve (in mm Hg). This method does not require the assessment of the systolic ejection time or the transvalvular flow, and the peak systolic gradient instead of the mean gradient may be entered into the formula. However, in the presence of tachycardia, the formula is less accurate because the percentage of time/minute in systole and diastole changes markedly at higher heart rates. In order to account for this, the result should be divided by 1.35 for heart rates >90 (Angel adjustment).

12. **b.** The Fick principle assumes that the rate at which oxygen is consumed is a function of the rate of blood flow and the rate of oxygen pick up by the red blood cells. In the cath lab, it is used to determine cardiac output by the difference in oxygen concentration in blood before it enters and after it leaves the lungs, and from the rate at which oxygen is consumed. Three variables need to be identified:

- Vo_2 consumption per minute using a spirometer (with the subject rebreathing air) and a CO_2 absorber
- the oxygen content of blood taken from the pulmonary artery (representing mixed venous blood)
- the oxygen content of blood from a cannula in a peripheral artery (representing arterial blood)

From these, cardiac output can be calculated:

$$CO = O_2 \text{ Uptake} / ([\text{Arterial } O_2] - [\text{Venous } O_2])$$

While considered to be the most accurate method for cardiac output measurement, Fick measurement is invasive, requires time, and the attainment of reliable oxygen samples. Quantitative ventriculography is a rather crude estimation of cardiac output and is infrequently used. Pulmonary artery thermodilution calculates cardiac output by quantifying a "temperature curve"; a small amount (typically 10 mL) of cold saline is injected into the pulmonary artery and the temperature a known distance away (6 to 10 cm) is attained, using the same catheter. Higher cardiac outputs will change the temperature rapidly, whereas lower cardiac outputs will change the temperature slowly. The technique is liable to gross errors unless certain requirements are strictly adhered to, and in certain clinical circumstances.

13. **d.** Mixed venous blood in a well patient at rest is about 75% saturated, which indicates that under normal conditions tissues extract 25% of the oxygen delivered. In general, any clinical condition which leads to an Svo_2 <60% threatens tissue oxygenation, and an Svo_2 <30% should be viewed as a medical emergency. True mixing of venous blood (in the absence of shunt) occurs in the pulmonary artery; therefore, slow aspiration from the distal lumen of a pulmonary artery catheter can provide a sample.

14. **e.** Other relative contraindications include decompensated heart failure, presence of left ventricular thrombus, acute coronary syndrome, mechanical aortic prosthesis, or endocarditis of left-sided valves. For all these reasons, ventriculography is more sparingly performed, especially given the myriad other noninvasive imaging options available.

15. **b.** The balloon should be inflated either in the terminal end of the inferior vena cava, or in the right atrium. In the femoral vein, the balloon or vein might be traumatized due to the relatively narrow diameter. The balloon should always be inflated before entering the right ventricle in order to reduce the risk of ventricular ectopy or free wall perforation.

16. **a.** The LAO projection is ideal for visualizing and "opening" the aortic arch, thereby delineating the origins of the innominate, left carotid, and left subclavian arteries. It is also useful for identifying the origin and extent of type A aortic dissection. The RAO view can be particularly useful when searching for aorto-coronary bypass grafts to the left coronary system.

17. **b.** Dyskinetic wall motion refers to paradoxical wall motion during systole. Aneurysmal dyskinesis is frequently appreciated after a transmural myocardial infarction and is a particular risk for development of mural thrombus. With time, dyskinetic injury will heal into akinetic scar.

18. **c.** Left aorto-coronary bypass graft usually originate superior and anterolaterally in the ascending aorta. The AL2 catheter is a good choice if the aortic root is dilated. In many cases, all grafts can be cannulated with a JR4. Both

the MPA and the LCB are useful in certain circumstances. The JL4 does not generally cannulate left-sided grafts.

19. **a.** Often, grafts to the RCA arise from the inferior aspect of the aortic root and descend aggressively down to the distal RCA or PDA. The JR4 is usually the default initial catheter for attempted cannulation of grafts, but in this instance it may be a poor choice. The JR4 is unlikely to cannulate in a coaxial manner, so injection into the ostium may lead to inadequate ("streaming") or absent filling. The MPB is often a good selection because of its modest primary bend, thereby aligning it well with an acute inferiorly angulated graft.

20. **b.** Usually, the location of the various grafts in relation to one another follows a predictable sequence. Grafts to the LCX are typically placed most superior, followed in succession inferiorly by grafts to the diagonal branches of the LAD, the LAD itself, and the RCA (see Figure 4-1).

21. **d.** The best view to assess LIMA to LAD anastomosis is 90° lateral view. In this view, the LAD lies below the sternum. Straight PA cranial is the best view for mid and distal LAD. Choice B is the best view to assess LMT, LAD, and left circumflex bifurcation. Straight PA caudal will best show the LMT, proximal LAD, and the left circumflex.

22. **d.** The best view to localize the origin or the presence of bypass grafts to LAD or left circumflex is the LAO 35° to 40°. The anterior and lateral border of the ascending aorta should be carefully reviewed frame by frame. The operator should account for each myocardial territory either by the presence of collaterals or by visible graft stump before concluding graft occlusion. For grafts to RCA, an RAO 35° to 40° view is best. Straight PA cranial or caudal is almost never used when performing aortography.

23. **d.** The best catheter for engaging an upward takeoff graft is usually AL2. This catheter should be formed in the distal ascending aorta and slowly pushed down to the level of interest. Subsequent clockwise or counterclockwise rotation should engage the grafts. At times once engaged the catheter must slightly be pulled back for better engagement. In order to disengage, the catheter should be pushed down and rotated so that it is no longer in the same plane as the ostium of bypass graft. For downward takeoff, we typically use Multipurpose B1.

24. **d.** Fluoroscopy and bony landmarks are extremely important and should be used for every case if a groin approach is undertaken. However, based on most recent large studies, the radial approach is the safest technique to reduce groin-associated complications. This approach is safe and has rarely

been associated with hand complications. In general, there is a learning curve associated with the radial approach. The use of ultrasound and micropunture needle can significantly decrease groin complications; however, it is associated with longer procedure time.

25. **d.** There has been conflicting data regarding the best method to reduce CIN. In general, the two most accepted methods to reduce CIN are hydration with normal saline and using as little contrast as possible. However, for patients at risk of CIN (diabetes, known chronic kidney disease, and history of CIN), a multimodality approach including *N*-acetylcysteine, sodium bicarbonate, and low-osmolar nonionic contrast in addition to biplane angiography to minimize contrast use is recommended.

26. **a.** The safest and most reliable method to establish hemostasis is manual compression. The use of vascular closure device in calcified, diseased arteries has been associated with dissections and high failure rate.

27. **b.** Perclose allows reaccess through side lumen if necessary. In our institution, Perclose has been the preferred device for coronary, structural, and peripheral interventions. However, this device has an associated learning curve. As noted in Chapter 9, data on closure devices are mixed. Our own analysis has shown Perclose to be slightly superior at least for patients undergoing coronary intervention.

28. **d.** The safest and most effective method to treat common femoral artery pseudoaneurysm is ultrasound-guided thrombin injection. With this technique, over 97% of common femoral artery pseudoaneurysms can be safely treated. Covered stent should rarely be used in the common femoral arteries because it is a bend region. Surgical correction is associated with morbidity. Ultrasound-guided compression may be effective for small pseudoaneurysm; however, it will rarely work for pseudoaneurysm over 2 cm.

29. **b.** In general, the safest approach when dealing with sheath-related dissection in the groin area is using the contralateral side to evaluate the extent of the dissection. In most cases once the sheath is removed, the dissection flap closes and no other intervention is necessary. In cases where there is hemodynamic compromise and the common femoral artery is involved, surgical approach is best tolerated. If surgery is not available, balloon angioplasty alone may be a reasonable option. In general, one should avoid stenting the common femoral artery.

30. **d.** Complications from closure devices occur in 0.5% to 1% of patients undergoing a diagnostic cardiac catheterization. It is important to remain vigilant for potential complications immediately after deploying a closure device as well as 1 to 2 weeks after the procedure when patients return for follow-up.

Intermittent claudication or acute limb ischemia occurs more commonly with collagen-based biosealant devices, whereas pseudoaneurysm or retroperitoneal bleeds can be seen with any closure device. Other potential complications not listed above include arteriovenous fistula and infection. The incidence of infection is higher with closure devices that leave foreign material at the arteriotomy site.

31. **False.** Only hemostatic pads should be considered with a 4-Fr. French sheath and selected devices with a 5-Fr. sheath (i.e., Perclose Proglide). However, closure devices are generally not necessary when using smaller French systems (4 or 5-Fr.) because manual compression is cost-effective and satisfactory from a patient perspective (i.e., short bedrest time and time to ambulation).

32. **e.** A knowledge of common causes of hypotension in the cath lab is essential. As a principle, identifying the task immediately prior to onset of hypotension often narrows the differential diagnosis (see Table 8.2). The patient in the clinical vignette is clearly in cardiogenic shock and this is the main cause of hypotension, but there are important potential contributing factors that need to be understood to treat this patient appropriately. Hypotension occurred immediately after two events: arterial access and sedation/intubation. Although a vagal reaction may occur as access is being obtained, this is usually transient and relatively benign, unlike this patient's clinical course. It is important to think of a retroperitoneal bleed as treatment would entail volume expansion (i.e., fluids and blood transfusions) as well as inotropic support. A retroperitoneal bleed in this patient is unlikely as hypotension does not occur immediately after obtaining arterial access. Depending on the rate of bleeding, it may occur late in the case or during recovery. Sedation and intubation causing loss of adrenergic drive is an important contributor to this patient's hypotension.

33. **d.** Profound hypoxemia in this patient occurred following endotracheal intubation. Although it is important to keep anaphylaxis to lidocaine in the differential diagnosis, there are no other clinical signs of anaphylaxis. Pulmonary edema may be a contributing factor, but it does not explain a sudden decrease in blood oxygen saturation. Tension pneumothorax and a right-to-left intrapulmonary shunt can be easily evaluated with fluoroscopy. This patient did not have a pneumothorax. The tip of the endotracheal tube was in the right main stem bronchus causing profound hypoxemia from a right-to-left intrapulmonary shunt.

34. **b.** The origin of both renal arteries from the lateral aspect of the aorta is variable. The right renal artery commonly originates slightly anterior and a shallow left anterior oblique projection may be best to identify the origin of both renal arteries. However, it is important to make adjustments for optimal visualization of each renal artery (i.e., the view that maximizes the length of the tip of the catheter). Occasionally, cranial or caudal angulation may be necessary to optimize visualization of the renal artery ostium.

35. **False.** Direct cannulation of a femoropopliteal synthetic vascular graft less than 6 months old should be avoided to decrease the risk of graft complications (i.e., bleeding or graft thrombosis). This patient's graft is 4 months old.

36. **c.** In patients with peripheral vascular disease, use of a micropuncture needle kit should be considered at the start of the procedure. The threshold for using a Doppler needle system (SMART needle) should be low in difficult access cases. In patients with calcified vessels, the common femoral artery can be accessed under direct fluoroscopic guidance.

37. **a.** In general, iliac arteries are best visualized using contralateral angulation. However, visualization of the pelvic arteries is often performed in the straight AP projection using a power injection. In cases of tortuous vessels or eccentric lesions, angulated views are necessary. The common iliac arteries are best visualized using contralateral angulation and the external iliac arteries may be best visualized using ipsilateral angulation.

Page numbers followed by *f* indicate figures; those followed by *t* indicate tables.